The Ketogenic Diet

A Treatment for Children and Others with Epilepsy, Fourth Edition

John M. Freeman, MD
Eric H. Kossoff, MD
Jennifer B. Freeman
Millicent T. Kelly

16pt

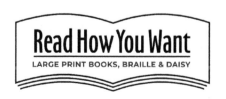

Read How You Want
LARGE PRINT BOOKS, BRAILLE & DAISY

Copyright Page from the Original Book

Visit our website at www.demosmedpub.com

Library of Congress Cataloging-in-Publication Data

The ketogenic diet : a treatment for children and others with epilepsy / John M. Freeman
... [et al.].—4th edition
    p.   cm.
   Previous ed. has title: The ketogenic diet : a treatment for epilepsy.
   Includes bibliographical references and index.
   ISBN-13: 978-1-932603-18-7
   ISBN-10: 1-932603-18-2
   1. Epilepsy in children—Diet therapy. 2. Ketogenic diet. I. Freeman, John Mark. II.
Freeman, John Mark. Ketogenic diet.

   RJ496.E6F69 2006
   618.92'8530654—dc22

                              2005031806

Special discounts on bulk quantities of Demos Medical Publishing books are available
to corporations, professional associations, pharmaceutical companies, health care
organizations, and other qualifying groups. For details, please contact:

Special Sales Department
Demos Medical Publishing
386 Park Avenue South, Suite 301
New York, NY 10016
Phone: 800-532-8663, 212-683-0072
Fax: 212-683-0118
Email: orderdept@demosmedpub.com

Made in the United States of America

06 07 08 09 10   5 4 3 2 1

TABLE OF CONTENTS

IMPORTANT NOTE TO READERS

This book introduces the ketogenic diet to physicians, dietitians, and parents of children with difficult-to-control seizures who might benefit from the treatment. The book is not intended to be an instruction manual. A book cannot take into account the specific needs of any individual patient. As with any course of treatment for epilepsy, a decision to try the ketogenic diet must be the result of a dialogue between parents and their child's physician.

THIS DIET SHOULD *ONLY* BE INITIATED under the supervision of a physician and a trained dietitian or nurse.

If you are reading this book, we assume that you are familiar with the basic descriptions of epilepsy and what they mean. This is not a book about seizures or about epilepsy. This is a book about one form of treatment for epilepsy—the ketogenic diet. If you wish to learn more about the condition called epilepsy, we suggest that you read the award-winning book *Seizures and Epilepsy: A Guide, Third Edition* by JM Freeman, EPG Vining and D Pillas, published by John Hopkins University Press.

OTHER TITLES BY JOHN M. FREEMAN, MD

Seizures and Epilepsy in Childhood: A Guide, Baltimore: Johns Hopkins University Press, 3rd Edition, 2003.

Tough Decisions: A Casebook in Medical Ethics, New York: Oxford University Press, 2nd Edition, 2000.

OTHER KETOGENIC DIET MATERIALS AVAILABLE

Introductory Video to the Ketogenic Diet. To order, send a written request and a check for $10.00 (shipping and handling) to: The Charlie Foundation To Help Cure Pediatric Epilepsy, 1223 Wilshire Blvd. #815, Santa Monica, CA 90403-5406. See www.charliefoundatio n.org for more information.

Additional copies of this book may be obtained from Demos Medical Publishing, 386 Park Avenue South, New York, NY 10016; (800) 532-8663; (fax) (212) 683-0118; orderdept@demosmed pub.com.

FOREWORD

On March 11, 1993, I was pushing my son, Charlie, in a swing when his head twitched, and he threw his right arm in the air. The whole event was so subtle that I didn't even think to mention it to Nancy, my wife, until a couple of days later, when it recurred. She said she had seen a similar incident. That was the beginning of an agony I am without words to describe.

Nine months later, after thousands of epileptic seizures, an incredible array of drugs, dozens of blood draws, eight hospitalizations, a mountain of EEGs, MRIs, CAT scans, and PET scans, one fruitless brain surgery, five pediatric neurologists in three cities, two homeopaths, one faith healer, and countless prayers, Charlie's seizures were unchecked, his development "delayed," and he had a prognosis of continued seizures and progressive retardation.

Then, in December 1993, we learned about the ketogenic diet and the success that Dr. John Freeman and Mrs.

Millicent Kelly had been having with it at Johns Hopkins Hospital as a treatment for kids with difficult-to-control epilepsy. We took Charlie there; he started the diet. Charlie has been virtually seizure-free, completely drug-free, and a terrific little boy ever since. He had to remain on a modified version of the ketogenic diet for a few years after being on the full diet for two years, but he goes to school and leads a normal, happy life. If we had had the information in this book 15 months earlier, a vast majority of Charlie's $100,000 of medical, surgical, and drug treatment would not have been necessary, a vast majority of Charlie's seizures would not have occurred.

The publication of the first edition of *The Epilepsy Diet Treatment* was supported by The Charlie Foundation so that other children and their parents and doctors who struggle with this problem can be informed about the ketogenic diet, as perfected at Johns Hopkins. We hope this book will help others decide whether the diet is a viable alternative to their current treatment, and we know that it will be a valuable guide once the ketogenic diet has begun.

Jim Abrahams, Director
The Charlie Foundation to Help Cure Pediatric Epilepsy

PREFACE

"Yuck!" was once the common response to the ketogenic diet. It was the response of parents and, indeed, of many physicians who did not have experience with the diet. The concept of a mere diet being able to control otherwise uncontrollable seizures seemed far-fetched to many back in 1994, when we reintroduced the ketogenic diet with the initial publication of *The Epilepsy Diet Treatment: An Introduction to the Ketogenic Diet.* Eleven years later, with the help of the first three editions, the ketogenic diet has become a widely accepted therapy for children with difficult-to-control seizures. It has won over skeptics and gained acceptance among both physicians and the public. A growing number of medical centers around the world are developing the expertise needed to administer the treatment successfully. The limiting factor in its use seems to be the lack of adequately trained dietitians, who are the prime ingredient in the diet's implementation and success.

Few new therapies in modern medicine have come to the fore in so short a time. Modern medicine treats epilepsy with pharmaceuticals, with anticonvulsant medications. Because it is based on food, the ketogenic diet is considered by many to be an "alternative therapy," but it is one of the few "alternative therapies" that has, through careful studies and demonstrated success, become a part of the mainstream medical treatment for epilepsy.

Research to understand how the diet works is once again active but, as discussed elsewhere in the book, has not yet brought extensive understanding. Perhaps the biggest advance in the ketogenic diet is the general acceptance that the diet *does* work. Efforts to discover *how* it works remain in progress.

Since the first edition of this book was published, a huge amount of new information has been generated on the ketogenic diet:

- New data from clinical studies and laboratory research have expanded our knowledge about many aspects of the ketogenic diet, including growth on the diet, weight gain, effects on serum lipid levels, and effectiveness of the diet.

- Experience with hundreds of new patients has deepened our understanding of the best approaches to helping children and their families cope with the limitations and restrictions of the diet.
- Feedback from many sources has been received—from conferences, publications, and private communications with neurologists, dietitians, and parents.
- New and improved menus have been developed, including some created by professional chefs whose children went through the diet. The ketogenic diet now is available in many countries throughout the world and has incorporated many ethnic foods.
- The needs of modern dietitians have evolved, and to meet these needs, instructions for calculating and managing the diet on a day-to-day basis have been revised.

- Ongoing laboratory research points to potential future improvements in ketone measuring techniques, and potential new ways to administer ketogenic diets effectively in a less restrictive manner.

The debate now taking place is not whether the diet is useful, but what place the diet should hold in the management of difficult-to-control seizures in children. Should it be offered only after a child has failed all available medications? After she has failed two medications? Should it be limited to children over 1 year of age? Will it work in adults? While we know of no reason why an adult should not attempt the diet, its efficacy and side effects in adults have not been widely studied. Is its usefulness limited only to those with epilepsy?

Even today, with all the new anticonvulsant medications that come on the market, many children still are burdened with difficult-to-control seizures. The ketogenic diet, although difficult to follow, if properly done, remains more effective than any of these new anticonvulsant medications.

It seems clear that, if the diet were a drug, companies would be promoting it as the treatment of choice for difficult-to-control epilepsy. Unfortunately, no companies are available to champion and promote the diet.

THE KETOGENIC DIET SHOULD *ONLY* **BE** USED under close medical supervision. The decision to use it should be the result of a dialogue between physicians and parents. It is rarely successful without the continuing support of an experienced physician and a knowledgeable dietitian.

The ketogenic diet is not the answer for everyone. But for some, it may result in a better quality of life, with fewer side effects, than any other therapy.

Many, many questions remain to be answered about the ketogenic diet. However, this new edition of *Ketogenic Diets* reflects the many advances in understanding that have taken place since the book was first published 11 years ago.

John M. Freeman, MD
Eric H. Kossoff, MD
Jennifer B. Freeman

ACKNOWLEDGMENTS

We are grateful to the many parents and children who have been treated at Johns Hopkins and have so willingly cooperated with our ongoing clinical research by collecting information, returning for follow-up, and giving blood. The data we have accumulated was only partially supported by research grants. Without your help, we could not have accumulated the knowledge about the diet and its effects that has converted many skeptics into believers and allowed the ketogenic diet to help so many children.

To the many physicians who have referred patients to the Johns Hopkins program and who have participated with and cooperated with our studies, we express deep appreciation.

We also want to acknowledge those parents whose phone calls have been met with busy signals, or who have been placed on hold for long periods of time, and those who have had to wait for days to have their questions answered. To all of you, we send our apologies and hope for your understanding.

Within weeks after a TV program about Charlie Abrahams and the ketogenic diet aired on *Dateline* in 1994, the small staff of the Johns Hopkins Pediatric Epilepsy Center responded to more than 5,000 inquiries. The innumerable continued phone contacts from parents who have brought their children to Johns Hopkins, and from those who are just interested in the diet, would have tried the patience of a less dedicated team. The close personal attention that has made the diet more acceptable to and more effective and manageable for many children could not have been accomplished without the staff's enduring talent and dedication.

We would specifically like to acknowledge and thank:

DR.EILEEN P.G. (PATTI) VINING, long time colleague and partner in this and many other endeavors to help children and families with epilepsy. She now directs the John M. Freeman

Pediatric Epilepsy Center at Johns Hopkins.

DIANA J. PILLAS, manager and coordinator-counselor of the Pediatric Epilepsy Center, whose tireless, indefatigable care and concern for parents and children with seizures or epilepsy has touched and improved untold numbers of lives.

PAULA L. PYZIK, who has collected, coded, and analyzed the information about children on the ketogenic diet and who has made it possible to finally provide data, not merely impressions, about many clinical facets of the diet.

We must, of course, acknowledge our gratitude to the Epilepsy Center's secretaries and staff, both past and present, who have done an amazing job juggling phone calls from parents who think their questions require an immediate answer and those whose calls have not yet been returned, while making appointments for children who needed to see us yesterday.

Last, all of this would not have come about without the commitment and dedication of Millicent T. Kelly, who retired as the dietitian of the Epilepsy Center at Johns Hopkins. It was through Millie that the wisdom of the diet was preserved through its years in the wilderness. It was her dedication that helped to revive interest in the diet and helped us to document its ability to improve the lives of many children.

SECTION I

OVERVIEW OF THE TRADITIONAL KETOGENIC DIET

CHAPTER ONE

EPILEPSY TODAY AND THE PLACE OF THE KETOGENIC DIET

A SEIZURE IS an alteration in behavior, consciousness, or movement due to an electrical discharge in the brain. Epilepsy is defined as having two or more seizures.

Seizures come in many forms, depending on where in the brain they start and how, and how rapidly, they spread. They can be the big shaking kind, termed *grand mal,* or they can be staring spells, termed *petit mal* or *absence* seizures. A seizure may be as simple as the dropping of the head to one side or as dramatic as crashing to the floor. Ten percent of all people will have a single seizure at some time during their lifetime; only 30 percent of those will ever have a second seizure. Some individuals will have recurrent seizures on occasion. Some even have them frequently. These frequently recurring seizures are called *epilepsy*. Epilepsy is not a disease; it is a symptom of a disruption in the electrical activity of the brain. It is like a short circuit, like static on your radio.

Epilepsy comes in many shapes and sizes:

- Children (and adults) with epilepsy may be otherwise normal; they may be teachers, workers, business people, and farmers. They may be your neighbor or friend. You may not even know they have epilepsy. People with epilepsy may be in college, doing very well. They may be athletes or even nerds.
- Children (and adults) with epilepsy may have mental retardation or motor dysfunction, termed *cerebral palsy.* They may have handicaps large or small.
- Most individuals with epilepsy can have their seizures completely controlled, in which case their

epilepsy may not be a handicapping condition.

- Some individuals have severe seizures that interfere with their quality of life. Some have additional intellectual or motor handicaps.

This book is about the ketogenic diet, a high-fat, low-carbohydrate, adequate-protein diet that is useful in controlling the seizures of many individuals whose seizures are handicapping and otherwise difficult to control.

After a single seizure, about a 30 percent chance exists of having a second seizure. On the other hand, a 70 percent chance exists that a child will be seizure-free for the rest of her life. For this reason, most neurologists do not start medications after just one seizure, except in very unusual circumstances.

Once a second seizure occurs, a 70 percent chance exists of a third seizure occurring. Unless the two seizures are very far apart in time, neurologists often start medications after the second seizure to try to prevent more seizures.

ANTICONVULSANT MEDICATIONS

All anticonvulsant medications are designed to help control seizures; they are not cures for the condition of epilepsy. Anticonvulsant medications usually are taken for several years, so that the brain can mature and the child will have a chance to "outgrow" the epilepsy.

For those children who continue to have seizures that affect their quality of life, medications are necessary and important. Twenty years ago, physicians had just a handful of medications to work with. In 2006, we have nearly 20 medications, double the number of only a decade ago.

Many of the newer medications have fewer side effects than the older drugs. However, many of these newer medications are not approved by the U.S. Food and Drug Administration (FDA) for use in children. This does not mean that they are unsafe or that they cannot be used in children. "Not approved" simply means that these drugs have not been sufficiently studied in children for the FDA to allow the drugs to be advertised for use in children. Once a medication has been approved for use in adults, the FDA controls the advertising of the medications, but physicians govern their use.

DESPITE ALL THESE NEW MEDICINES, it is not clear that a child with difficult-to-control epilepsy is much better off now than 20 years ago. The same percentage of children who didn't respond to medicines in the past aren't responding now.

After a second seizure (which results in a diagnosis of epilepsy), about two-thirds of children have their seizures controlled by the first medication used, usually without major side effects.

If side effects do occur, or the seizures are not controlled, another anticonvulsant is tried. Twenty to twenty-five percent of children who did not respond to their first medication will respond to the second or third drug.

Sadly, 10 to 15 percent of children with epilepsy do not seem to respond to any medications. Many recent studies in both children and adults have shown that, if the first two or three drugs don't work, doctors and parents should not waste time testing a fourth or fifth drug, but should move on to other options. Typically, this is where the ketogenic diet is currently used. Perhaps, in some cases, it should be used even earlier.

SURGERY

After even one drug has failed, neurologists often think about brain surgery as an option. Thinking about surgery is not the same as intending to operate but, in some cases, surgery is an important option. If seizures are coming from one area of the brain, *and* if that area of the brain is available for removal without causing brain dysfunction, *then* epilepsy surgery may be the best option for controlling seizures.

Surgery might not be an option if:

- A single area is not clearly found, despite testing with electrodes placed on the brain.
- Seizures are coming from many different regions of the brain.
- Seizures are coming from an important area involving movement, language, or memory.
- The child has other medical issues that make surgery too risky.

When surgery is not an option and medications fail, children experiencing seizures are left with few choices. These include the ketogenic diet and vagus nerve stimulation (VNS). Depending on their doctor, one of these therapies is typically recommended. At Johns Hopkins, we often recommend the ketogenic diet first. Others may recommend the diet only after a VNS is unsuccessful.

Our experience is that a VNS is often a help, but rarely a cure. It is probably less commonly a cure than the ketogenic diet.

WHERE DOES THE KETOGENIC DIET FIT IN?

The ketogenic diet commonly is used after two or three medications have failed, and if surgery seems unlikely to help. At Johns Hopkins, we are using it earlier in the course of epilepsy than at most other centers. We have seen some dramatic results with the diet, for even the toughest of seizure cases. The diet can be given to young infants, teenagers, and even adults in some cases. Side effects are generally low and, if they occur, are often reversible without having to stop the diet.

Multiple studies have shown that half of all children who have failed multiple medications will have more than a 50 percent decrease in their seizures on the ketogenic diet (Table 1.1). About a third will have a greater than 90 percent improvement. About 10 percent become seizure-and medication free. When this occurs, everyone is thrilled. It is very hard to predict who will respond in this way to the diet without at least a 1-month trial period.

Every child and every family who embarks on the ketogenic diet dreams of a total cure. Sometimes, their dream comes true. Megan, a highly motivated 12-year-old with a supportive family, was able to "cure" her seizures after 2 years on the diet. Here is a letter written by Megan's parents after she had been on the diet for just 6 weeks:

 TABLE 1-1

Outcomes of the Ketogenic Diet: Johns Hopkins Patients, 1998

Number Seizure Control Initiating and Diet Status	Time After Starting the Diet		
	3 months	6 months	12 months
Total N = 150			
Seizure-free	4 (3%)	5 (3%)	11 (7%)
>90%	46 (31%)	43 (29%)	30 (20%)
50–90%	39 (26%)	29 (19%)	34 (23%)
<50%	36 (24%)	29 (19%)	8 (5%)
Continued on diet	125 (83%)	106 (71%)	83 (55%)
Discontinued diet	25 (17%)	44 (29%)	67 (45%)

MEGAN'S STORY

DEAR DR.FREEMAN,

I want to share with you and your team the wonderful changes in Megan's life since she has been on the ketogenic diet.

As you remember, we were having very serious and frightening prospects as a family.... Megan's seizures, which we called "stares," were out of control in spite of using three drugs. She was experiencing so many an hour that she was regressing both in school and in her personal skills. She would be unable to remember what she had been doing prior to a "stare," and therefore had difficulty staying focused on tasks—whether keeping her place in her reader or even dressing herself, or just remembering what she went to get in another room.... Being only 10 years old, she was very frightened because she was not able to stop "staring," and children teased her. She cried because she would wake up at night and not realize she was in her own bedroom. She also described many auras in which she reported seeing flashing lights and people's faces changing colors....

We could not increase the Depakote level because of the side effects to her stomach. She was taking Mylanta three times daily just to coat her stomach to tolerate the

Depakote. And still her stomach hurt, resulting in poor appetite—which ... had reduced her weight to the tenth percentile for her age group. This constant concern over her eating patterns and small consumption had also created tension in our family over meals.

The ... seizures also resulted in her ... sleeping at least 12 to 13 hours out of each 24, including sleeping an hour at school midday.

As a result of all these physical changes, the disorder now took Megan's social life. Since she had to go to bed so early, she couldn't go to church or ... school functions. On Saturdays, she could play only in the morning because she would sleep in the afternoon. Spending the night with a friend became out of the question because she didn't get enough sleep—which increased the "stares."

Her neurologist felt surgery would have to be considered—that Megan would likely become worse. He recommended Johns Hopkins

Hospital and your team. And so we came, expecting to have to take the chance of even losing her life in the surgery, in order to give her the chance of improving quality of life—and save the very essence of our spirited, enthusiastic, loving child.

Due to the complexity of Megan's neurological situation, you did not recommend surgery, but offered her something incredible—a diet! You told Megan she could use her strength to turn down sugar from her friends and to stay on her diet. We will never forget how her little face lit up when you said "no surgery."

Her life has literally turned around from that day. She has been very dedicated to learning about labels with sugar, preparing foods, etc., and is determined to stay on her diet.

It has been and will be worth the extra time it requires to plan and prepare the meal plans. She has had only two "stares"—one the day of dismissal from the hospital, the other at school when she began decreasing the Dilantin level.

She has really had a learning spurt. Her reading teacher ... tested Megan and ... confirmed the improvement in reading already! Megan is thrilled to be promoted to a harder reader. Her memory also improved, and she is being assigned more difficult words. She is choosing her clothes and dressing herself with little supervision from me. She is going to slumber parties!

Family and friends say over and over they can tell how well she is doing. Her thoughts are well connected in conversation. Megan says, "I'm so much better than before I went to Baltimore. I can remember things now. I'm doing great!" In short, she is alert and happy.

After seven and a half years of dealing with frequent and frustrating medication changes with varying side effects, this diet is a fantastic alternative. I will not complain! This Christmas was our most joyous *since the first Christmas after she was born.*

—MH

The diet was not easy. Megan's family had to learn step by step how to organize life around it for 2 whole years. Megan cried the time she won a spelling bee in her class and the prize was a pizza, of which she could take not even a single bite. "I shared it with all of the class, but I couldn't have any myself," she later recalled. Megan's own motivation, as well as her supportive family, was key to making the diet a success. The fact that the diet was 100 percent successful was highly motivating and its own reward.

Megan remained on the diet for 2 years and has now been off the diet for many years—seizure-free and medicine-free. Despite structural damage to her brain, which had caused the epilepsy and a mild hemiparesis, she has just graduated from high school and plans to go on to more studies. Asked if the diet was worth it, Megan replied, "It gave me my life back."

Megan's story is dramatic, and grateful parents have written many similar letters. Articles about children with 100 percent success stories have appeared in newspapers and periodicals around the country, with headlines such as "Michael's Magical Diet," "Cured by Butter, Mayo, and Cream," and "High-Fat and Seizure Free." These are the glowing reports of the dramatic success that the diet can achieve.

CASEY'S STORY

DEAR DR.FREEMAN:

Ever since I picked up that little yellow book, The Ketogenic Diet: A Treatment for Epilepsy, *I have wanted to write you a letter to let you know how much I appreciate your work. This is long overdue, but I wanted to share our story with you.*

The past two weeks, I have watched my 4-year-old son take swimming lessons. As I watched him splash and play in the water, I started thinking back over the past 15 months.

It all started in April. It was a normal evening at home, when all of a sudden my son started staring into space. I didn't panic until he stopped breathing. As the ambulance raced towards our house, he started making small jerking movements with his legs. It was at this point that I realized he was having a seizure. Although the hospital is only 15 minutes from home, I felt that we had been in the back of the ambulance for 2 hours. He passed all of his "tests," and we were sent back home. On the way to the pediatrician's office the following day, he began having another seizure in his car seat. This one was more violent than the first—he was completely limp when the EMT pulled him from the car. Again, we raced to the hospital, this time determined not to leave until we found what was wrong with our son.

We had been in the emergency room almost 3 hours when the nurse came out to say she had contacted the pediatrician. We were given the name of a pediatric neurologist and told to call and make an appointment. We told her we were not leaving the hospital until we knew what was wrong with our child. As she left to make a call to the pediatrician, our son began having a third seizure, this one worse than the other two. Having seen it, she could describe it to the doctor, and we were transferred to a larger hospital with a special ward for children.

That night was full of testing—CT scan, MRI, EEG, all kinds of blood work. It was a nightmare. After a night of absolutely no sleep, we met with the pediatric neurologist. She introduced herself, and said that Casey had a mild case of epilepsy and that he would probably outgrow it. She gave us a prescription. A few days later, he began having a different type of seizure—drop attacks. When he began having more and more of them, I did some research and discovered that they are one of the most difficult seizure *types to control. After 8 weeks, we switched to Topamax, then to phenobarbital, Depakote, Keppra, then Trileptal, then Zonegran. It was a never-ending trip to the pharmacy.*

Casey was a zombie. His color was gone. His former permanent grin was reduced to an occasional little smile. He started wetting his pants. His constant staring was interrupted only by the 25 to 30 drop attacks he had every day. We finally decided that nothing could be lost by seeking another opinion.

At the University Hospital, we met another pediatric neurologist, who was the first person to mention the amazing treatment we are now experiencing. The dietitian recommended your book The Ketogenic Diet: A Treatment for Epilepsy. Several days later, we were admitted to the hospital. On Monday, we started his fast ... By Thursday, his drop attacks had started to dwindle and we could take him home. In 2 weeks, I noticed that his personality was coming back. He smiled and laughed like he used to. He was interested in everything again. My little boy was coming back.

After 12 weeks, he went 3 whole days with zero drops. A cheating spell gave us a few bad days, but before long, he was back to being seizure-free. I almost felt that I could stop holding my breath ... If we can keep him from cheating, I believe he will overcome his illness.

I know we have a long way to go with the diet—and I have no idea what the future will hold. But as I watched him jump into the pool all by himself today, I thought about how far he has come in the past 4 months. As his little blond head popped back up from under the water and he looked at me and grinned, he said, "Mommy, I did it! All by myself!"

I think that we are in the middle of a miracle.

Thank you for your work in childhood epilepsy—and thank you for the book that taught me so much about the diet that is giving my son his life back.

—LM

DEFINING SUCCESS

Unfortunately, the ketogenic diet does not result in a success story for everyone. Almost half of all children who start the diet stop during the first year. Some stop because, despite the medical and support team's best efforts to "fine-tune" the diet (see Chapter 8), and despite the family's diligent efforts, the seizures have not improved sufficiently to make their efforts worthwhile. Some discontinue because of illness, noncompliance, or because the diet is "just too hard."

For example, Jay[1] was a 15-year-old whose seizures started at age 9 years. In 6th grade, he had so many dizzy spells and seizures that he missed 77 days of school. In 7th grade, he was

---

[1] Jay's name and those of some others throughout the book have been changed to protect their privacy.

taking 16 pills per day and still missed 108 days of school. He had brain surgery in which his temporal lobe was resected, but the seizures returned. Jay and his family then decided to try the ketogenic diet.

Jay's goal, like that of many teenagers, was to be able to drive. For this, he needed to be 100 percent seizure-free. On the ketogenic diet, he fell short of this goal—he was nearly, but not completely, seizure-free. Five months after starting the diet, Jay's mother reported that he "lives on sausages, eggs, and choked-down heavy cream at every meal." "We are always in the kitchen ... cutting, cleaning, weighing," his parents wrote. "We never go out to eat anymore or have pizza at home. At Thanksgiving, the whole family ate eggs."

Jay's seizures were much improved, and his medications were reduced, but without being seizure-free, Jay believed that he would never be able to drive and therefore the diet was too much trouble. The diet was discontinued after about 9 months.

With so much improvement in seizure control, was Jay's experience with the diet a success? Well, yes and no. His seizures were markedly decreased and his medications were reduced. However, his major reason for undertaking the diet was to become 100 percent seizure-free so that he could drive. Since he wasn't able to reach this goal, the diet was—for him—a failure.

Perhaps, using current knowledge, Jay's diet could have been fine-tuned to further improve seizure control. A more supportive and creative family might have found ways to go out for meals and spend less time in the kitchen, to make life on the ketogenic diet closer to normal. But Jay's family could not or did not. From the perspective of his Hopkins support team, Jay's experience with the diet was a failure—not because it didn't completely eliminate his seizures, but because we thought (in our optimistic fashion) that it could have been a success but for variables beyond our control. Ultimately, however, it is the child and the parents who must define the diet's "success" or "failure."

AT FIRST, WE DIDN'T GO OUT, even to my parents'. I was afraid of temptation, of making my son sad for what he couldn't have. But he missed the socializing. He said, "How come we never go out anymore?" I told him, "You couldn't order anything on the menu anyway." He said, "I could get ice for my ginger ale!" Now, we go to a restaurant and take his meal with us. He tells the waitress, "I'm on a special diet so just bring me ice, please."

—CC

If the diet is working, most families find ways to integrate it into a happy, active life. Ingenuity, flexibility, good humor, and lack of self-pity go a long way toward making the diet acceptable to both the child and the family.

WHEN SHOULD THE DIET BE USED?

The ketogenic diet is not the treatment of choice for people who have experienced only one seizure, or even for those who have had only a few seizures. If seizures can be successfully controlled by a single medication, without side effects, then most will find that the rigors and sacrifices required by the diet are not worthwhile.

However, the diet should *not* be reserved only for children who have failed all possible medications. We see far too many children who have been tried on multiple medications for several years before they are offered the ketogenic diet. *The diet should not be considered the treatment of last resort.*

Similarly, it should *not* be used merely because a child's parents don't find medications "natural."

The ketogenic diet *should* be tried earlier in the course of treatment for the child whose myoclonic-akinetic seizures are difficult to control with medications, and perhaps in the child with Lennox-Gastaut syndrome. The diet is less likely to work in the presence of a structural lesion, but still can be given a try before surgery. Its role in the early treatment of infantile spasms is not known. Chapter 5 contains more information about these reasons to start the diet.

Sylvia is a good example of our uncertainty about who is a good candidate for the ketogenic diet. Brought to us when she was 18 months old, Sylvia had suffered constant seizures, despite good trials of medications, ever since she had experienced a very near sudden infant death syndrome (SIDS) episode at 3 months of age. She did not see, hear, or respond. She had not even cried for more than a year. Her mother asked us to try the ketogenic diet.

When asked what she hoped the diet would accomplish, Sylvia's mother replied that the baby would be easier to care for if the seizures were under better control. This seemed reasonable, so Sylvia was admitted for the diet. After fasting and 2 days of ketogenic formula, Sylvia started to cry. Her mom burst into tears of joy at the sound.

On the fifth day of the diet, Sylvia smiled. Her seizures decreased markedly, but did not come under control for almost 9 months. After a year and a half on the diet, Sylvia was sitting and playing. Later, she started standing and interacting—drug-free and seizure-free. She remains severely mentally and physically impaired, but there *was* a little girl in there.

Even with seizures under fairly good control, medication may affect children's alertness and mental clarity, impairing their ability to learn and reach their full potential. Therapy for epilepsy is often a balance between seizure control and medication toxicity.

The point at which an individual's seizures are deemed out of control, or side effects are considered unacceptable, varies from person to person and from family to family. When we studied letters that parents wrote about their expectations at the time of their children's ketogenic diet initiation, we found that they varied considerably. One hundred seizures a day is clearly too many, but are three seizures a month too many? Some children and families consider it a victory to limit seizures to one a week, while others consider one seizure every 2 months an intolerable state of affairs.

Varying degrees of sedation, hyperactivity, and learning disabilities may be acceptable in exchange for seizure control. But, what if you could control seizures without such side effects? This is a question asked by many parents. Could my child learn better, faster, and more easily without the toxicity of the medication? Would her behavior and attention improve if she weren't on anticonvulsants? How can you tell when a child cannot be taken off medication without the chance of recurrent seizures? The net result is that many children and their parents look beyond currently available medications for a satisfying solution to seizure treatment.

When children are admitted for the ketogenic diet, we routinely ask them to write us a bit about what they want the diet to achieve and what they would consider success. This serves two purposes. It helps parents to focus on what is important to them, and it provides the medical team with a benchmark to measure against to show how close a child is to meeting parental expectations when he returns for follow-up.

When we reviewed one hundred parent expectation letters, we found:

- Although seizure and medication reduction was the most common desire, 90 percent of families wanted something else as well.
- The parents' most common additional desires were improved learning, better alertness, fewer injuries, and happiness for their child.
- Most parents were very realistic and did not expect complete freedom from seizures or medication.
- Parents whose children were on the diet and did achieve good seizure control and improved learning were nearly always able to remain on the diet.
- The diet either met or exceeded the parents' initial goals for seizure improvement in 57 percent of families.
- The diet either met or exceeded the goals for medicine reduction in 44 percent.

- The diet either met or exceeded the parents' initial goals for improved learning and alertness in 59 percent.

MICHAEL IS DRUG-FREE and *seizure-free! He was singing "Jingle Bells" last week, but changed the words to something like this:*
Jingle Bells, I'm a special kid,
Cause I'm on the magic diet.
Oh, what fun it's gonna be
To not have seizures anymore!

Isn't that something? We laughed so hard, we cried. Like so many Americans, my faith lay in drugs or surgery ... My feelings now cannot be adequately expressed. The meals do take time to prepare, and there are other difficult things to get through, but its working! IT'S WORKING! Michael is a different child being off the drugs. More alert, more physical, more talkative (boy, is he!). More everything. I feel we now have a whole child. All because of a diet. I would not wish this diet on my worst enemy, but I would wish it on every child with uncontrolled seizures. It could be the beginning of a whole new life.

—EH

I CALL IT THE "VOODOO DIET." My son remembers when he was on the medication. He calls it "when I was bad" or "when I couldn't control myself." He used to rock back and forth, flip the light switch fifty times, make loud noises, bite himself, bite other people, put his hand in a flame, you name it. His seizures were fairly well controlled; he was only having maybe one a month or every 6 weeks. His doctor said, "This kid's seizures are pretty much under control on the medicine. What more do you want?" What I wanted was for my boy to get his old, sweet personality back.

He has had no seizures or medication for a year and a half on the diet. He likes himself now. He is content with who he is. I can hardly believe it. Anyone who sees him can hardly believe he is the same kid. I am certainly glad that

I tried this diet, despite the fact that it ties you to the house and it ties you to the meals. I hate the diet. I mean, the minute it's over, I'm going to bomb my food scale. But it has helped my son so immensely that I can't hate it too much.

—CC

For many parents, the ketogenic diet, which does not have the cognitive and behavioral side effects of anticonvulsant medications, offers a chance—though sometimes an unattainable dream—of seeing their child free of medications and seizures. For many parents, it is as important to see their child free of medication as to see them free of seizures. For others, like the family of Jay described earlier, the ketogenic diet is not considered a success unless seizures are completely eliminated. Even among those who discontinue the diet, however, most find the attempt at the diet worthwhile because, as they often say, "at least we know that we tried."

CHAPTER TWO

WHAT IS THE KETOGENIC DIET?

The ketogenic diet is a medical treatment for controlling seizures by switching a body's primary metabolism to a fat-based energy source, rather than utilizing glucose.

The ketogenic diet simulates the metabolism of fasting. When a fasting person has burned up all his glucose stores, after about 24 to 36 hours, his body then begins to burn stored body fat for energy. A person on the ketogenic diet derives energy principally by burning the fat in the diet, rather than from the more common energy source, carbohydrate (glucose). But, unlike fasting, the ketogenic diet allows a person to maintain this fat-burning, partially dehydrated metabolism over an extended period of time.

The body obtains energy from three major food sources:

- Carbohydrates—Starches, sugars, breads, cereal grains, fruits, and vegetables
- Fats—Butter, margarine, oil, and mayonnaise
- Proteins—Meat, fish, poultry, cheese, eggs, milk

Carbohydrates comprise approximately 50 to 60 percent of an average American's daily caloric intake. The body converts carbohydrates to glucose, which is burned by the body to produce energy. When the supply of glucose is limited, the body burns fat for energy. If insufficient fat is present, then muscle is burned, compromising good health. The body maintains only about a 24-hour supply of glucose and, once glucose is depleted, the body automatically draws on its backup energy source—stored body fat.

In the absence of glucose, fat is not burned completely, but leaves a residue of "soot" or "ash" in the form of ketone bodies that build up in the blood. The ketogenic diet is designed to maintain this buildup of ketone bodies in the blood by forcing the body to burn fat as its primary source of energy, instead of glucose. The ketones that are left from the burning of fat are *beta-hydroxybutyric acid* and *acetoacetic acid.* The betahydroxybutyric acid can be used by the liver and by the brain as a source of energy. Acetoacetic acid is excreted in the urine and imparts a sweet smell to the breath that has been likened to pineapple.

When ketone levels are large enough, as indicated by a simple urine test, it is said that the body is "ketotic" (pronounced key-tah´-tic) or in a "state of ketosis." Ketosis also is evidenced, as mentioned above, by a fruity, sweet odor to the breath. In the presence of large levels of ketone bodies, seizures are frequently controlled.

The ketogenic diet is high in fat and low in carbohydrate and protein. It is made up of about 85 percent fat, 10 percent protein, and 5 percent carbohydrates. Calories are restricted to about 75 percent of the standard amounts recommended for a child based on age, but this is increased if the child is underweight and may be lowered if a child is overweight. Although not proven, we believe that a child must be close to ideal body weight for the diet to work best and for ketosis to be strongest. Fluids are also restricted to 80 percent of the daily requirement.

Traditionally, the diet is initiated slowly over 3 days, after a 48-hour period of fasting (a limited amount of carbohydrate-free fluids are allowed during this period). Details of the Johns Hopkins approach to starting the diet are discussed in more detail in Chapter 7.

THE KETOGENIC DIET is a rigid, mathematically calculated, doctorsupervised therapy. This diet should only be attempted under the close supervision of a physician and dietitian.

FOODS

Common, but carefully selected, ingredients are used in meals that a child can eat while on the ketogenic diet. With the help of a dietitian and careful calculations, the diet can be adapted to many foods and many cultures around the world.

The diet also can be started as a liquid formula for bottle-fed infants and children with a gastrostomy feeding tube. For the parents of these children, the diet can be fairly easy to administer since compliance is not an issue, and the formula tastes as good as regular baby formula.

Some young children are on a combination of formula and solid foods, depending on their eating abilities.

Sample meal plans

A more detailed discussion of sample meal plans is presented in Section 5, Chapter 16. The following is an example of what 2 days of meal plans might look like for a child on the diet:

Breakfast #1	Breakfast #2
Scrambled egg with butter	Bacon
Diluted cream	Scrambled eggs with butter
Orange juice	Melon slices
	Vanilla cream shake

Lunch #1	Lunch #2
Spaghetti squash with butter	Tuna with mayonnaise

and Parmesan cheese

Celery and cucumber sticks

Lettuce leaf with mayon-
naise

Sugarless Jell-O with
whipped cream

Orange diet soda mixed
with whipped cream

Dinner #1	Dinner #2
Hot dog slices with catsup	Broiled chicken breast
Asparagus with butter	Chopped lettuce with may-onnaise
Chopped lettuce with may-onnaise	Cinnamon apple slice with butter topped with vanilla ice cream
Vanilla cream popsicle	

Ketogenic diet menus depend on the desires of the child and the imagination of the parent. One breakfast might include a mushroom omelet, bacon, and a cream shake, another a special keto-recipe cold cereal. Keto cereal was invented by the mother of a child who missed eating his bowl of cereal in the morning. The creative mother crumbled keto cookies (recipe below) in a bowl and poured cream over them. This made excellent cold cereal that satisfied her son.

KETO COOKIES OR KETO CEREAL

Ingredients:

2 egg whites

1 teaspoon cream of tartar

1 small package of flavored sugar-free Jell-O™

A few drops carbohydrate-free flavoring, if desired

Beat the egg whites until stiff. Stir in cream of tartar and Jell-O™. Spoon onto a nonstick cookie sheet, about 1 tablespoon per cookie.

Bake at 325° for 6 to 8 minutes or until brown.

Makes 20 cookies. 1 serving=2 cookies.

For cereal, crumble into a bowl and add cream.

By identifying the four main food groups of the diet—protein, fruit or vegetable, fat, and cream—in each of these sample menus, you can begin to understand how the diet is constructed. This will be explained in greater detail in Chapter 12.

MYTHS AND MISUNDERSTANDINGS

Contrary to the belief of some parents, the ketogenic diet is not "all natural," "holistic," "organic," or "pure." The ketogenic diet is a means of using food to treat seizures in children and perhaps in adults as well. The diet may be more effective for some forms of seizures than are current medications. It definitely is a substantial intrusion on a family's life. However, physicians and families weigh the difficulties and benefits of the ketogenic diet compared to medications and to seizures, and try to do the best thing for each child.

The ketogenic diet is not completely free of side effects. In general, the ketogenic diet is better tolerated than most medications, and it has fewer potential side effects. However, it does have side effects. The major side effects seen with the diet are: lack of weight gain, *slightly* decreased growth, *somewhat* high cholesterol, constipation, kidney stones, and acidosis. All are reversible without having to stop the diet. Details of side effects will be discussed in Chapter 9.

The diet is not the best choice for everyone. Emma's family, for example, thought *any* diet would be better than giving their daughter drugs. They believed that medications were unnatural and had side effects, so they tried to keep Emma off anticonvulsants. Emma had tried gingko and St. John's wort, and she had made several trips to chiropractors and hyperbaric oxygen treatment centers. Nothing had helped her seizures. After a long discussion with neurologists at Johns Hopkins, though, Emma's parents began to recognize that, although the diet was perhaps an option, medicines, if effective, would be much simpler! An anticonvulsant medication was started, and Emma became seizure-free after 3 weeks. She never had to go on the ketogenic diet.

The ketogenic diet requires a lot of commitment and a lot of work. Medications are easier to use, if they are effective without substantial side effects. Even for families who become expert in preparing the diet and organizing their lives around it, the ketogenic diet is a big undertaking. Thus, physicians usually recommend that an individual with seizures should try one or two medications before turning to the diet. Anticonvulsant medications are far easier to use and, if they work, they are probably a better choice than the diet.

A modified Atkins diet, which will be discussed in Chapter 15, is somewhat easier than the traditional ketogenic diet, but it is still not easy.

Common Misunderstandings

- *"He will be seizure-free."* Some children do become seizure-free, but only about 1 in 10. Half of children who try the diet do not receive enough benefit to make it worth continuing.
- *"She will get rid of all those poison medicines that have side effects and are not even approved for use in children."* This is a result to be desired, but it is not a reality for everyone. First, a child has to have good control of her seizures. Only

then can doctors can try to decrease or eliminate medicines.

- *"We will just try it for a few weeks and, if it doesn't work, we'll go back to medications."* We ask each family for a 3-month commitment. After starting the diet, it takes 3 months to "fine-tune" it, finding the correct amounts of calories, finding the correct spacing of the meals, and getting both the child and the parent accustomed to this new lifestyle. Initiating the ketogenic diet requires too many changes and commitments on the family's part, and too much commitment from the whole keto team, to have someone not give it a proper chance.

CHAPTER THREE

HISTORY OF THE KETOGENIC DIET

Fasting has been used as a treatment for seizures and epilepsy since biblical times, and it is mentioned again in the literature of the Middle Ages. However, it wasn't until the 1921 American Medical Association convention, at which Rawle Geyelin, a prominent New York pediatrician, reported the successful treatment of severe epilepsy by fasting, that interest in this approach to treatment began to reawaken. Geyelin cited the case of a "child of a friend," age 10, who "for 4 years had had grand mal and petit mal attacks which had become practically continuous." At Battle Creek, he came under the care of an osteopath (Dr. Hugh Conklin), who promptly fasted him, the first fast being one of 15 days. Several subsequent periods of feeding then fasting occurred. "After the second day of fasting," Geyelin reported, "the epileptic attacks ceased, and he had no attacks in the ensuing year." Geyelin reported seeing two other patients, also treated by Dr. Conklin, who, after fasting, had been seizure-free for 2 and 3 years. He further reported that he had fasted 26 of his own patients with epilepsy, 18 of whom showed marked improvement and two of whom remained seizure-free for more than 1 year. Dr. Geyelin stated that the best length of fasting was 20 days. This was the first American report of the benefits of fasting on epilepsy.

The following year, Dr. Conklin published his belief that epilepsy was caused by intoxication of the brain by toxins coming from the Peyer's patches of the intestine. He had developed his "fasting treatment" program in order to put the patient's intestine at complete rest. He stated, "I deprive the patient of all food, giving nothing but water over as long a period of time as he is physically able to stand it.... Some will fast for 25 days and come to the office one or more times every day for (osteopathic) treatment...."

> **WE NOW KNOW** that epilepsy has nothing to do with the Peyer's patches of the intestine, but we have learned that fasting seems to curtail seizures.

Dr. William Lennox, considered by many to be the father of American pediatric epilepsy, relates Conklin's fasting treatment to the origin of the ketogenic diet. According to Lennox, who later reviewed Geyelin's records, long-term freedom from seizures occurred in 15 of 79 of Geyelin's fasted children (18 percent).

It is also of historical interest that the father of Hugh Conklin's patient, HLH, reported by Geyelin, was Charles Howland, a wealthy New York corporate lawyer. The boy's uncle was Dr. John Howland, Professor of Pediatrics at the Johns Hopkins Hospital and director of the newly opened Harriet Lane Home for Invalid Children at Johns Hopkins in Baltimore. In 1919, Charles Howland gave his brother $5,000 to find a scientific basis for the success of the starvation treatment in his son. These funds were used to create the first

American laboratories to study fluid and electrolyte balances in fasting children. Although these studies shed light on fluid and electrolyte balance in children, and were the start of the investigational careers of many great pediatric physicians, Howland and his team were unsuccessful in finding how starvation helped to control seizures.

During the early 1920s, when only phenobarbital and bromides were available as antiseizure medications, reports that fasting could cure seizures were exciting and promised new hope for children with epilepsy. These reports set off a flurry of clinical and research activity at many centers.

The early 1920s was also an era during which early investigations were made into understanding the metabolic basis for diabetes, the inability of the body to metabolize glucose, and the often-fatal ketoacidosis that accompanied diabetes. A 1921 review article about diabetes and its dietary management stated "acetone, acetic acid, and ß-hydroxybutyric acid appear (even) ... in a normal subject (caused) by starvation, or a diet containing too low a proportion of carbohydrate and too high a proportion of fat. [Ketoacidosis] appears to be the immediate result of the oxidation of certain fatty acids in the absence of a sufficient proportion of 'oxidizing' (dissociated) glucose." In diabetic ketoacidosis, the inability to burn glucose leads to exceedingly high levels of blood glucose, with resulting dehydration of the tissues and chemical imbalances that lead the patient to coma and sometimes to death. These effects clearly are not occurring with either starvation or the ketogenic diet, in which glucose is restricted.

THE DISCOVERY OF THE KETOGENIC DIET

The first article suggesting that a diet high in fat and low in carbohydrate might simulate the metabolic effects of starvation and its effects on epilepsy was published in 1921. Wilder, its author, proposed that, "the benefits of fasting could be ... obtained if ketonemia was produced by other means.... Ketone bodies are formed from fat and protein whenever a disproportion exists between the amount of fatty acid and the amount of sugar. It is possible," Wilder wrote, "to provoke ketogenesis by feeding diets which are rich in fats and low in carbohydrates. It is proposed to try the effects of such diets on a series of epileptics." The calculation of such a diet, and the effectiveness of Wilder's proposed "ketogenic" diet, was reported in 1924, from the Mayo Clinic, by Peterman. Peterman's diet used 1g of protein per kilogram of body weight in children (less in adults), restricted the patient's intake of carbohydrates to 10 to 15g per day, and the remainder of the calories were ingested as fat. The individual's caloric requirement was calculated based on the basal metabolic rate plus 50 percent. This is virtually identical to the ketogenic diet that is used today.

Of the first 17 patients treated by Peterman with this new diet, 10 (59 percent) became seizure-free, 9 on the diet alone. Four others (23 percent) had marked improvement, two were lost to follow-up, and one discontinued the diet. The following year, he reported 37 patients treated over a period of 2.5

years: 19 (51 percent) were seizure-free, and 13 (35 percent) were markedly improved. These initial reports were rapidly followed by others from many centers. The currently used protocol for calculating and initiating the ketogenic diet is well discussed by Talbot in 1927.

Reports of the effectiveness of the diet appeared throughout the late 1920s and 1930s. In these reports, subjects varied and patients were followed up for varying lengths of time. As shown in Table 3.1, early reports of the diet showed 60 percent to 75 percent of children generally had a greater than 50 percent decrease in their seizures, 30 percent to 40 percent of these had a greater than 90 percent decrease in the seizure frequency, and 20 percent to 30 percent had little or no seizure control.

The ketogenic diet was widely used throughout the 1930s. When diphenylhydantoin (Dilantin) was discovered in 1939, the attention of physicians and researchers turned from the mechanisms of action and efficacy of the diet to the new anticonvulsants.

A new era of pharmacologic treatment for epilepsy had begun. Compared with the promise of the medications, the diet was thought to be relatively difficult, rigid, and expensive.

As new anticonvulsant medications became available, the diet was used less frequently. As fewer children were placed on the ketogenic diet, fewer dietitians were trained in its rigors and nuances. Therefore, the diet was often less precise, and so less ketogenic and less effective than it had been in previous years.

In an effort to make the ketogenic diet more palatable and less rigid, a form of the diet was developed using medium-chain triglyceride (MCT) oil. This oil was more ketogenic and allowed larger portions of food, but children on the MCT diet often suffered from nausea, diarrhea, and bloating; therefore, despite the decrease in seizures, parents often found the side effects unacceptable and gave up. During the 1980s, Schwartz and her colleagues in Oxford, England, conducted the only comparative trial of the various diets that had been developed. Testing the classic ketogenic diet, the MCT diet, and a "modified" MCT diet, their study (Table 3.2) showed that 41 percent of patients had a greater than 90 percent seizure reduction. No one diet was superior to others. More children found the MCT diet unpalatable, and diarrhea and vomiting were more common on the MCT diet.

TABLE 3-1

Reports from the Literature on Seizure Control Using the Ketogenic Diet*

Author	Year	Number of Patients	Seizure Control > 90%	Seizure Control 50–90%	Seizure Control < 50%
Peterman	1925	36	51%	35%	23%
Helmholtz	1927	91	31%	23%	46%
Wilkens	1937	30	24%	21%	50%
Livingston	1954	300	43%	34%	22%
Kinsman	1992	58	29%	38%	33%
Huttenlocher (MCT)	1971	12	—	50%	50%
Trauner (MCT)	1985	17	29%	29%	12%
Sills et al. (MCT)	1986	50	24%	20%	26%

*Representative studies.

MCT=medium-chain triglyceride diet.

Experiences such as these led to the widespread opinion that diet treatment for epilepsy did not work or was very difficult to tolerate. Many doctors also believed that parents and children would not be strong or rigorous enough to comply. Medicines, and the promise of even more effective medicines on the horizon, were disincentives to using the ketogenic diet.

TABLE 3-2

Comparison of Clinical Responses to Various Ketogenic Diets

	Reduction in Seizure Frequency		
	> 90%	50–90%	< 50%
Diet (59 individuals)*			
Classic 4:1 (N = 24)	11	11	2
MCT (N = 27)	10	11	6
Radcliffe (N = 12)	5	3	4
N studies (N = 63)	26 (41%)	25 (40%)	12 (19%)

Adapted with permission from Schwartz et al., *Dev Med Child Neurol* 1989; 31:145–151.

*Some who failed one diet were tried on another.

Even today, although we understand considerably more about the neurochemistry and neurophysiology of seizures and epilepsy, we do not understand the factors that initiate a seizure. We do not know the mechanisms by which seizures are stopped, or what inhibits some from spreading. We know some of the neurochemistry and physiologic events that accompany the electrical discharges of single cells, and we are only beginning to study the interactions of cellular populations. We know some of the chemistry and physiologic effects of medications, but we still do not know how anticonvulsant medications work.

THE START OF THE MODERN ERA

In 1993, Charlie Abrahams, age 2, developed multiple myoclonic seizures, generalized tonic and tonic-clonic seizures, which were refractory to many medications. As his father Jim Abrahams wrote in the foreword to this book, "thousands of seizures and countless medications later," when physicians were unable to help, he began to search for answers on his own and found reference to the ketogenic diet and to Johns Hopkins. Charlie was brought to Johns Hopkins, where the diet was still prescribed. After starting on the diet, Charlie's seizures were completely controlled, his EEG returned to normal, his development resumed, and he no longer suffered the side effects of medication.

Charlie's father wanted to know why no one had told him about the diet before. He found references to the high success rates discussed previously and determined that this information should be readily available so that other parents could become aware of the ketogenic diet. Creating the Charlie Foundation, Charlie's father, a filmmaker and fundraiser, used his talents to expand the use and awareness of the ketogenic diet. He funded the initial publication of this book. Charlie's story was covered in national magazines and on national television, starting with the news magazine show *Dateline,* further raising awareness of the diet. After the *Dateline* program about Charlie aired in 1994, the 1,500 copies of the first printing of this book immediately sold out.

When we told him that Johns Hopkins could not conceivably handle the number of patients who would want the diet after the *Dateline* show, Jim and the Charlie Foundation funded five pediatric epilepsy centers to come to Johns Hopkins for a meeting to plan a joint protocol to re-evaluate the efficacy of the diet in children failing modern medications. Over the next few years, the Charlie Foundation underwrote conferences to train physicians and dietitians from medical centers nationwide. Many medical centers began to use the diet.

Jim created the made-for-TV film "First Do No Harm" dramatizing the ketogenic diet. He also filmed our educational efforts about the diet for parents, dietitians, and physicians. He produced videos about the diet for parents, families, children, and for physicians, and made the tapes available to those audiences. Meanwhile, Nancy Abrahams spent tireless hours coaching and helping other parents during their difficult times with the diet. She spoke at countless parent meetings and conferences, and she provided support for those in need.

After Charlie remained seizure-free for 2 years, he was allowed to come off the diet, but several months later had a few further seizures. He resumed the diet in January 1996, and again became seizure-free on a modified form of the ketogenic diet. Charlie has now been seizure-free, medication-free, and off the diet for years.

Without Jim and Nancy's persistence, and their dedication to making knowledge of the diet available to other parents, to physicians, and to the public, the ketogenic diet would likely not have been "rediscovered" so dramatically and would not have experienced the resurgence in popularity it now enjoys.

The history of this rapid expansion in use and awareness is well described by Wheless, who concluded in 1995 that the ketogenic diet compares favorably with other new treatments for epilepsy in children. The diet offers a far greater chance for seizure control than any of the anticonvulsant medicines developed in the past 50 years. In 2005, more than 70 countries around the world offer the diet.

Prospective studies evaluating the effectiveness of the ketogenic diet are available. A 1998 multicenter study of 51 children who averaged 230 seizures per month before starting the diet (Table 3.3) documented that almost half (45 percent) remained on the diet for 1 year (a measure used in trials of medication to assess both effectiveness and tolerability) and almost half of those (43 percent) remaining on the diet (Column B) were virtually seizure-free. Eighty-three percent of those remaining on the diet for 1 year had better than a 50 percent decrease in their seizures.

 TABLE 3-3

Outcomes of the Ketogenic Diet: A Multicenter Study

	Number (%) of Those on Diet by Intention to Treat			
	A 6 months	B 12 months	C 6 months	D 12 months
Initiated Diet N = 51	N = 34 (66%) on diet	N = 23 (45%) on diet	N = 34 (66%) on diet	N = 23 (45%) on diet
> 90% sz. control	N = 14 (41%)	N = 10 (43%)	N = 14 (27%)	N = 10 (20%)
(No. seizure-free)	(6)	(5)	(6)	(5)
50–90%	N = 12 (35%)	N = 9 (39%)	N = 12 (24%)	N = 9 (18%)
< 50%	N = 8 (24%)	N = 4 (17%)	N = 8 (16%)	N = 4 (8%)
Discontinued diet	N = 16	N = 27	N = 16	N = 27
Patients missing	N = 1	N = 1	N = 1	N = 1

Reproduced with permission from Vining, Freeman et al. *Arch Neurology* 1998; 55:1433–1437.

This multicenter study also shows the difficulties of comparing new studies with older ones, which used a different approach to reporting their outcomes. If you look at this same multicenter study from a different angle, and include all of those children that the centers "intended to treat," meaning everyone who was started on the diet even if they only remained on it for a day or a week, then, as is shown in columns C and D, the same 45 percent of the children remained on the diet for 12 months. But only 10 (20 percent) of those starting on the diet had better than 90 percent seizure control at 1 year, and an additional nine children (18 percent) had a 50 to 90 percent decrease in seizures.

This newer "intention to treat" approach to reporting clinical trials of treatment gives a better concept of the chance of a treatment being effective. If we "intend to treat" a child with the ketogenic diet, the chance of decreasing that child's seizures by more than 90 percent are one in four, according to this methodology.

Since that study in 1994, we have started hundreds of children on the diet at Johns Hopkins. The outcomes of 150 consecutive children are shown in Table 3.4. Before starting the diet, these children averaged more than 600 seizures per month and had been on an average of more than six medications.

TABLE 3-4

Outcomes of the Ketogenic Diet—Johns Hopkins 1998

Number Initiating and Diet Status	Seizure Control	Time After Starting the Diet			
		3 months	6 months	12 months	3–6 years
Total N=150	Seizure-free	4 (3%)	5 (3%)	11 (7%)	20 (13%)
	>90%	46 (31%)	43 (29%)	30 (20%)	21 (14%)
	50–90%	39 (26%)	29 (19%)	34 (23%)	24 (16%)
	<50%	36 (24%)	29 (19%)	8 (5%)	18 (16%)
Continued on diet		125 (83%)	106 (71%)	83 (55%)	18 (12%)

Reproduced with permission from Freeman et al. *Pediatrics* 1998;102:1358–1363.

As Table 3.4 shows, even among children who could not be helped by modern anticonvulsant medications:

- Twenty-seven percent had their seizures controlled or virtually controlled after 1 year on the ketogenic diet: 7 percent were completely free of seizures, and 20 percent had a greater than 90 percent reduction.
- Half (50 percent) had a 50 percent or better decrease in their seizures.

It is notable that virtually all those remaining on the diet for 1 year had at least a 50 percent decrease in seizures. Those who had less than a 50 percent reduction often decided that the diet was too much trouble and discontinued it. It is also noteworthy that most children who had success with the diet had shown some success during the first 3 months. The degree of success might improve after 3 months, but if a 50 percent decrease in seizures did not occur during that time, it was less likely to occur in subsequent months.

The results appear as good as those from an earlier era, despite starting with children who have failed six—often new—medications and who were having an average of 600 seizures per month.

COMPARE THESE RESULTS with the fact that, if a child's epilepsy has not been controlled with the first two medications used, that child has only a 20 percent chance of being controlled with any further medication.

What is even more amazing is that 3 to 6 years after starting the diet, 13 percent of these 150 children were seizure-free, and another 14 percent had only infrequent seizures. Most of these children had also been able to discontinue their anticonvulsant medications.

We even have children that have stayed on the ketogenic diet for over 6 years. Most are seizure-free or nearly so, and many are medicationfree. Over time, they have found the diet relatively easy to do.

IN JANUARY, DANIEL HAD HIS FIRST TONIC-CLONIC SEIZURE .... In the months since then, he has had thousands of seizures. Drop attacks, "jerk" episodes, staring episodes, and more tonic-clonic seizures. I stopped counting when he hit 70 in any particular day. We met our doctor, who from the beginning told me that the ketogenic diet was certainly an option, but she wanted to try medication first.

Try medication we did! Topamax, Dilantin, Ativan, Keppra, Klonapin, and Zonagram, two of which caused nasty rashes...I had a zombielike child on my hands who was still seizing. And things got worse. I pulled him out of day-care and quit working.... I settled down into what I thought would be my life, with no hope of getting back my once bright, shining, happy, and intelligent little boy. I thought about this diet some more....

I met the dietitian. She asked me, "Do you think you can get him to drink whipping cream? If not he'll have to eat more butter." My stomach lurched. After measuring out his first meal (which took 45 minutes) I cried like I've never cried before. But somehow we got through it, and the next morning he had only five seizures. Five!!! The next day was even better.

He has been on the diet 20 days now. He has not had a seizure in 2 weeks. I know that you've heard stories like ours before. I know that we are one of the lucky ones. I am writing to say thank you for helping me to get my son back.

—NA

CHAPTER FOUR

HOW DOES THE KETOGENIC DIET WORK?

We know that the body is able to burn fats as a source of energy instead of its usual glucose, and that the brain is able to use the ketone bodies left over from fat burning as its own energy source. It appears that high level of ketones are associated with better seizure control, and we know that, in some individuals, even small amounts of carbohydrates can quickly break the ketosis and may result in seizures. We also know that in some children seizures can be completely controlled on the diet, and those children may after a time slowly discontinue the diet, often with no return of the seizures.

However, while ketones suppress seizures and carbohydrate interferes with this suppression, at present we do not know the mechanisms involved.

Understanding the mechanisms requires ongoing laboratory investigations. Understanding how the diet works will also require more information about seizures and epilepsy and, at present, we know remarkably little about either.

THEORETICAL BASIS OF THE KETOGENIC DIET

Although the short answer to the question, "How does the ketogenic diet work?" is, "We don't really know yet," the longer answer to the question is that a number of alterations of brain metabolism occur when an individual or an animal is fasting, has restriction of caloric intake, or is in ketosis. These potential mechanisms have recently been reviewed in the book *Epilepsy and the Ketogenic Diet* by C.E. Stafstrom and J.M. Rho (Humana Press, Totowa, NJ, 2004).

Ketone bodies, the hallmark of the ketogenic diet, are built up as a result of the incomplete burning of fats in the body. Ketones have a sedative and an appetite-suppressing effect. Some popular weight-reduction diets that feature very low calorie levels and low carbohydrates also produce ketosis. The appetite-suppressing effect of ketosis explains why these diets can be followed without the dieter's feeling too hungry.

Ketones also have an anticonvulsant effect. Small amounts of sugar, as, for example, when a child whose seizures are well controlled on the diet eats a cookie, may cause seizures to occur, even if urinary ketones are not clearly affected.

Although the concentration of ketones in the blood is clearly far more important than those in the urine, ketones are still measured in the urine for convenience. If no ketones are present in the urine, we know that the diet is not going to work. But, even if the ketones in the urine are high, we sometimes find that the diet can be made even more effective using a higher ratio of fats to protein and carbohydrates, or with fewer calories.

It seems apparent that, although the appearance of high ketone levels in the urine may predict good seizure control, measuring the urine levels of ketones is not always accurate. We are probably on the verge of finding that three to four plus ketones in the urine appear to be necessary for good seizure control, but they are not sufficient for such control.

In the early studies of diabetes, it was found that the hallmark of diabetes was sugar in the urine. Early diets were designed to decrease the sugar in the urine. The sugar content in the blood (like serum ketones) could be measured, but required a large amount of blood and was expensive. Gradually, less expensive and easier ways of measuring blood sugar were developed. Today, individuals with diabetes measure their own blood sugar with a finger prick and a glucose meter, and adjust their diet or insulin intake depending on the results.

Measuring ketones in the urine is inexpensive and easy, but it does not give a clear indication of the ketone levels in the brain, where the seizures occur. Sampling the brain is not possible; the ketone levels in the blood are a much closer approximation of the ketone levels in the brain than are those in the urine. However, sampling blood for the measurement of its ketone content is expensive and it does require a needle stick.

Our study correlating blood BOH (ketone bodies) with urinary ketones and seizure control suggested that blood levels of greater than 4mmol/L correlated best with seizure control. Urinary ketones of 4+or greater were found when the blood level exceeded 2mmol/L. Therefore, the urine should test at 4+ketones, but higher levels than that cannot be measured using ketogenic dipsticks. In the last edition of this book we concluded that 3+to 4+urine ketones are frequently necessary, but not necessarily sufficient to achieve optimal seizure control in children on the ketogenic diet. Unfortunately, the current apparatus for measuring blood ketones is not sufficiently reliable for home use, so we still test urinary ketone levels. But, in the future, when a reliable method of easily and cheaply measuring serum ketones at home is available, we will be close to the potential ability to titrate the diet to produce the necessary levels of serum ketones, if that proves to be the critical factor in controlling seizures.

Will that improve our ability to control seizures? Perhaps. It is probable that the ketogenic diet will, in the next several years, also be titrated by the patient or family to achieve specified amounts of serum ketones.

Acidosis is an increased amount of acid (pH level) in the blood. Ketone bodies are acids and therefore cause acidosis. Several other chemical mechanisms exist by which the human body produces acidosis. The body has many ways to compensate for the presence of ketones to maintain a normal pH balance. Acidosis is one of the factors that influences the threshold for some seizure types, such as absence seizures.

Acidosis may be one of the metabolic participants facilitating seizure control in the ketogenic diet but, because the body quickly compensates for acidosis to readjust its pH balance, acidosis is unlikely to be the major determinant of the diet's success.

Dehydration was part of the original water diet used by McFadden that ultimately led to the development of the ketogenic diet. Although fluids traditionally are limited during the diet, the role, if any, of dehydration in seizure control is unclear.

It is known that administering excess water can provoke seizures, probably due to acute dilution of the intracellular sodium level. Indeed, this was one of the methods used by physicians in the past to provoke seizures for observation. However, this in no way indicates that dehydration would prevent seizures by raising the body's sodium level. Normal kidneys do an excellent job of maintaining the body's chemical balance.

Another misconception about fluid intake is that fluid dilutes the urinary ketones, thereby negating the effects of the ketogenic diet. Increased water intake certainly results in urine that is more dilute. If the body's production and excretion of ketones is constant, the concentration of ketones in the urine (and therefore the strength of the urinary ketone test) will depend on the child's water intake. This diluted urine does not, however, necessarily reflect the level of ketones in the blood and brain.

None of the individual mechanisms discussed here will in isolation lead to seizure control, because the body can compensate for each of them. Acidosis corrects itself in 1 to 2 weeks, and the pH of the blood then remains normal throughout the remainder of the diet. The rest of the body rapidly compensates for changes in the water and electrolyte content of the brain.

The real effectiveness of the diet probably lies in other influences on metabolism.

Glucose is the preferred energy source for the brain during normal metabolism. Although the fetus and newborn are able to exist on a metabolism of fats, the brains of children and adults burn glucose almost exclusively. Does the ketogenic diet enable the brain to revert to this more primitive form of metabolism? There is some suggestion that a diet high in certain fats that produce particular ketone bodies, particularly ß-hydroxybutyrate (BOHB), may alter the chemistry of brain's cell membranes and thereby the sensitivity of certain transmitter sites. Clearly, more research is needed to explore the mechanisms by which the ketogenic diet achieves its dramatic results.

We have learned from recent research in animals that:

- Cerebral energy reserves are increased by chronic ketosis.
- Ketosis alters the metabolism of glutamic acid (an excitatory amino acid).
- ß-Hydroxybutyric acid, while not directly anticonvulsant, may affect aceto-acetate and acetone levels in the brain, and these do have anticonvulsant effects.
- Caloric restriction of itself may underlie the anticonvulsant effects of the ketogenic diet. This has been shown in animal studies using artificially created seizures.
- The ketogenic diet elevates the levels of norepinephrine, an inhibitory neurotransmitter that may play a role in the antiepileptic effects of the ketogenic diet.
- A high-fat diet may elevate polyunsaturated fatty acids (PUFAs),

which are modulators of neuronal hyperexcitability.

Perhaps Eagles and Baugh best summarized our current state of knowledge when they wrote: "In terms of the breadth of its anti-ictal (and anti-epileptic) efficacy, the Ketogenic Diet seems to stand alone. Its effectiveness argues ... for a role in altering fundamental metabolic processes as a key to the mechanism(s) by which the diet, caloric restriction, and starvation alter seizures and epilepsy."

In other words, many research projects are underway to discover the reasons for the clinical effectiveness of the diet. Outcomes research has stimulated basic research. Because the diet has been shown to work, investigators are now asking, "How does it work?" "What is its mechanism of action?"

THE NEED FOR RESEARCH

In the early 1960s, Dr. H. Houston Merritt, co-discoverer of Dilantin and then director of the Neurologic Institute at the Columbia Presbyterian Medical

Center in New York, told his residents that his discovery of Dilantin as an effective anticonvulsant was a major setback to the understanding of epilepsy. At the time the effectiveness of Dilantin was discovered, in the late 1930s, many people were investigating brain metabolism in epilepsy and beginning to study the mechanisms by which the ketogenic diet stopped seizures.

Since the discovery of Dilantin, however, efforts have been directed toward finding other drugs that would be equally effective, and few investigators have gone back to look at the basic mechanisms by which the ketogenic diet alters the brain's metabolism. However, since the reemergence of the diet during the past few years, all of that is changing. Studies using mice are showing that feeding a ketogenic chow can induce ketosis in the animals and can raise the animals' threshold for seizures. Other investigators are infusing BOHB and decreasing the animal's seizures. These first attempts to measure the effects of BOHB on the brain of laboratory animals may lead to an understanding of how the diet works and how it affects seizures and epilepsy.

Using new imaging technology, such as positron emission tomography (PET) and single photon emission computerized tomography (SPECT) scans, and with advancements in magnetic resonance imaging (MRI) spectroscopy, we can now study the human brain in action and the chemical and metabolic changes that rapidly take place during changing conditions, such as seizures. We are hoping to study the brain metabolism of those individual children who are having frequent seizures under conditions of starvation and during initiation of the ketogenic diet, analyze acute changes in metabolism, and evaluate longer-term changes in brain energy metabolism with continuation of the diet. We hope to compare children for whom the diet is unsuccessful with those in whom the diet stops seizures. We hope to then compare the alterations in brain metabolism that take place when a small dose of glucose is given to a child in whom the diet controls seizures. Through studies such as these, we hope to improve the understanding of why and through what mechanisms the ketogenic diet works.

While it may be distressing not to know the mechanisms by which the ketogenic diet works, this fact is far less distressing when one realizes how little we know about epilepsy and about how anticonvulsant medications work. One place to begin comprehending the depths of our ignorance is with some of the most commonly asked questions:

- Why does my child have epilepsy? In more than 70 percent of children, we don't know. Most seizures are "idiopathic" in origin, a fancy word for "we don't know where it comes from or why." We do know that epilepsy from known causes is more difficult to control than idiopathic epilepsy.

- Since he has epilepsy, why do his seizures occur once per hour (or per day, or month)? We don't know why individual seizures occur. Although we know some factors, such as fatigue, excitement, illness, fever, may predispose a child to a seizure, we rarely know what causes a seizure to occur at a specific time. We do not even know how these factors alter the threshold for seizures or what causes a seizure to stop on its own, as it usually does.

- Why are some seizures just focal jerking, while others spread to generalized tonic-clonic seizures? Why do some seizures involve staring spells and others a sudden drop attack? Little is known about the mechanisms by which the electricity of seizures spreads throughout the brain. We do not understand the directions of that spread, which determine the clinical manifestations of the seizure. We do not understand why one child's seizure threshold is lower than another's.

- Why do some children's seizures respond to a single medication, while others are not responsive to any anticonvulsant medication? Little is known about how the various anticonvulsants work. While we know many of the actions of older medications, such as phenobarbital and phenytoin (Dilantin), we still do not fully understand how they act to prevent seizures.

If we understand so little about the causes underlying seizures and the mechanisms of the medications commonly used to treat epilepsy, it should not be surprising that we do not understand the mechanisms of action of an old-fashioned diet. However, it is clear that, whatever the diet's mechanisms of action, these are likely to be different from the mechanisms of action of the drugs we currently use. The wide variation in the diet's effectiveness in varying seizure types, and its action across varied ages, suggests that its basis of action will be different than most current anticonvulsant drugs. If and when we understand how the ketogenic diet works, then perhaps we also will understand more about epilepsy itself.

USE OF THE KETOGENIC DIET: A PHYSICIAN'S VIEW

Pediatric neurologists are aware of the ketogenic diet. Some remain skeptical, and some quite negative, yet they are at least somewhat familiar with the treatment. Many other physicians and many adult neurologists, however, are still not aware of the diet or remain unbelievers.

Fortunately, during in the past 5 years, more and more pediatric neurologists are able and willing to implement the ketogenic diet, and an increasing number are starting children with difficult-to-control seizures on it far earlier in the course of treatment. An individual does not have to fail six medications before trying the diet.

Every patient and physician hopes that the next anticonvulsant pill or combination of pills will help, but the fact remains that if a child has failed two medications used appropriately and in combination, only a 15 to 20 percent chance exists of controlling that child's seizures with the addition of *any* of the new medications. The new medications may decrease the frequency of seizures in adults (in whom these drugs are tested), but few give more than a 50 percent decrease in seizures, and complete control is rare. The chance of dramatic success using the newer medications is even less in the difficult-to-control populations. Using more than two drugs simultaneously in any patients dramatically increases the side effects of the drugs. Therefore, the addition of a third or fourth medication is only likely to result in a child who is toxic from medications and who has continuing seizures.

The ketogenic diet is a lot of trouble. But, if it works, if it decreases seizures by more than 50 percent or if it allows a substantial decrease in medication toxicity, it not only becomes tolerable, but the words "amazing," "fantastic," and "a miracle," can be loudly heard from the parents of children for whom it has been successful.

THE KETOGENIC DIET TODAY

Information on the nutritional content of almost all food is readily available. Information on processed foods, if not shown on the label, is available from the manufacturer upon request. However, the initiation of the diet requires a lot of work on the part of parents as well as dietitians. Success requires patience, persistence, care, and faith on the part of the whole team: the physician and the dietitian, as well as the parents. The medical community has learned to distrust alternative and nutritional therapies as a whole. But this distrust, too, may pass. The medical community can look back and judge the history of anticonvulsant medications—their efficacy and side effects—and compare them to the efficacy of the ketogenic diet.

With the knowledge embodied in this book and the convenience of computer calculations, we hope that physicians and dietitians will regain a familiarity with the benefits of the ketogenic diet and begin to use it earlier and more frequently in the course of treating pediatric epilepsy.

CHAPTER FIVE

IS MY CHILD A CANDIDATE FOR THE KETOGENIC DIET?

The ketogenic diet is potentially appropriate for almost any child with difficult-to-control seizures. We usually try at least two medications to control the seizures before considering the diet.

DOES THIS MEAN THE DIET WOULDN'T BE HELPFUL EARLIER?

Definitely not, and we suspect the opposite. In some cases, the diet may be considered before two medications have been tried, depending on the type of seizures and the judgment of the physician. But since most types of seizures can be controlled with only one medication—without side effects—this is better than changing your whole lifestyle with the diet. Therefore we usually suggest trying one or two medications before trying the diet.

Your child may be a candidate for the diet if:

- He has failed two or more drugs used appropriately
- He has severe side effects from the medications
- He has infantile spasms, which usually respond poorly to medications
- He has other seizure types with many "drop" spells, such as the Lennox-Gastaut syndrome or Doose syndrome
- He has tuberous sclerosis, schizencephaly, lissencephaly, or other major congenital malformations of the brain that are associated with seizures
- The child is very retarded, is fed by gastrostomy tube, or is very young and bottle-fed, in which cases the diet may be easier to use and more effective than trying medications.

The diet is appropriate for children who have difficulty with the side effects of medications, even if those medications are effective in controlling seizures. When compared to many anticonvulsants, especially those of the older generation (e.g., phenobarbital, phenytoin [Dilantin], divalproex sodium [Depakote], carbamazepine [Tegretol]), the diet has fewer, milder, and more easily reversible side effects. Less information is available about the effectiveness of the newer medications in children and about their side effects than is available for the ketogenic diet.

There are reasons why the diet isn't used first, before any medications. No doubt it is easier to take a pill than to measure every gram of food and change an entire family's lifestyle. Also, many physicians are not comfortable with the diet; many have been told by drug-company representatives that a new drug is "very effective" for a child's particular seizure disorder. They aren't told that the testing was done in adults and that the drug hasn't been tested in children. And they aren't told that "very effective" means that, in the study, the medication decreased the seizures by 50 percent in only 30 percent of the subjects—a smaller percentage of improvement than that noted for the diet.

Nothing is worse than seeing for a second opinion a child who has failed more than 10 medications over many years, and who was never offered the ketogenic diet as an option. Research shows that if a child still has uncontrolled seizures after good trials of two or three medicines, he is unlikely to gain good seizure control on any future medicines.

DO YOU EVER START TREATING A CHILD'S SEIZURES WITH THE KETOGENIC DIET RATHER THAN WITH MEDICINE?

Rarely! The ketogenic diet (and even the Atkins diet discussed later) is difficult and requires a major commitment from the family and from the child. If parents and children haven't struggled for a time with seizures, medication, and side effects, then the diet may seem too difficult. But on occasion...

SANDRA WAS A 5-YEAR-OLD with new onset frequent complex partial seizures. Her older brother Charlie had been on the ketogenic diet for 4 years, having come to see us after years of difficult-to-control seizures that didn't respond to any medications. Charlie had had a dramatic response to the diet, and the family wanted to try the diet with Sandra before other medications were tried. Since Sandra's parents had lots of experience with the diet, Sandra was started and did just as well as her brother. Their previous experience made the change in lifestyle much easier to handle.

HOW LONG DOES IT TAKE TO SEE IF THE DIET WILL HELP?

We ask each family to commit to 3 months on the diet, so that we can fine-tune the diet to the needs of the child. However, some children respond quickly and completely. Families see these "miracle" cures on TV and in the newspapers and expect their child will come to the hospital and leave seizure-free. This does happen, but only in a minority of our patients. After fasting, some children have no more seizures and are seizure-free within days and off their medications in weeks, *but that is not the rule.*

About 10 percent of the children become seizure-free on the diet and 25 percent have only rare seizures. Unfortunately, we cannot identify who will be our ideal patients and who will do less well. You just have to try the diet and see. Children of all ages and of most seizure types can respond.

SPECIAL DISORDERS

Certain neurologic conditions do extremely well on the diet and, while not extensively studied, show enough promise to be tried in additional children.

Infantile spasms

Children with infantile spasms are among the most difficult to treat. The frequent head and body drops are refractory to most medications and are frequently associated with mental retardation. Treatment with ACTH has serious side effects. Vigabatrin, also shown to be effective, is not currently available in the United States. We found that nearly half of 23 children with infantile spasms we treated with the ketogenic diet had a 90 percent or better response, improvement on EEG, and better development by 6 months. Children treated with the diet before 1 year of age or before three medications had been tried did better. With this success, perhaps the diet should be attempted as the first treatment for spasms.

Myoclonic-astatic (Doose) epilepsy

In this disorder, children between the ages of 3 and 5 years often present with the sudden onset of head-drop seizures and occasionally cognitive decline. It is similar in many respects to the Lennox-Gastaut syndrome. Traditional medicines are useful only occasionally. We have used the ketogenic diet in a small number of these children with occasionally dramatic success. This is another condition which deserves further study.

Tuberous sclerosis complex

In a small study of children with tuberous sclerosis, half the children had a greater than a 90 percent decrease in their seizures on the diet. Here again, the ketogenic diet is proved useful and deserves further study.

Glucose-1 transporter deficiency

In this very rare condition, the molecule that allows glucose to cross into the brain to be used as fuel is missing. Because the brain cannot receive adequate glucose, fat makes sense as a better alternative fuel. The highfat ketogenic diet makes a major difference in the functioning of these children and is considered the therapy of first and only choice for them.

IS THERE A BEST AGE TO TRY THE DIET?

Younger children have a slightly greater chance of doing well on the ketogenic diet than do older ones. Younger children often can maintain high ketosis for long periods, and compliance is less of a problem. For this reason, infants may be an ideal group for the diet.

WHAT ABOUT ADOLESCENTS AND ADULTS?

Many centers tell parents that it is impossible for a teenager to stick with the diet. Our small study of adolescents found that compliance among the adolescents was very good, seizure reduction was similar to younger children, and side effects were low. Most of our teenagers were very motivated, having often dealt with years of bad seizures, and they were willing to make the commitment the diet requires. They should not be discouraged from trying the diet.

Few adults have been studied, but the small number studied appears to have the same rates of compliance and the same outcomes as have been reported in children. Clearly, more extensive studies are needed in adults and in each of these populations. The Atkins diet, which has been widely used for weight loss, may provide seizure control and, in adults, may be less restrictive than the classical ketogenic diet. More information about the Atkins diet is presented in Chapters 15 and 17.

INTELLIGENCE

The level of a child's intelligence is not a criterion for selecting appropriate candidates for the diet. Some of the most dramatic successes have occurred in the most profoundly handicapped children. Other successes have occurred in children with normal intelligence.

However, it is important for parents to carefully assess their goals and expectations before starting the diet. Parents may believe that their child's substantial intellectual delay is due solely to their medications and that, if they could only get their child off medication, everything would be back to normal. Such parents are likely to be disappointed.

The diet is intended primarily to control seizures. Decreasing and discontinuing medications is only a secondary goal. Improving intellect is a hope and a desire, but that is not what the ketogenic diet is designed to do.

CHAPTER SIX

TWENTY QUESTIONS ABOUT THE DIET

Q *My child loves pizza and ice cream. Eating is an important part of our family life. How could we ever go on the diet successfully?*

A If you are creative, you can find a way to adapt and still follow the diet. Pizza? Try a grilled tomato or eggplant slice topped with cheese—this becomes a ketogenic pizza.

Ice cream? No problem! The cream in the diet can be frozen into scoops or popsicles, flavored with allowed sweeteners and baking chocolate, vanilla, or strawberries. The kind of pizza or ice cream your child is accustomed to having may seem unimportant when a "magic diet" helps to get rid of seizures!

Your child can go on the diet successfully because both of you want to cure the seizures. Much, perhaps most, of the diet's success depends on your positive attitude and persuasiveness as a parent. If a parent does not have a positive attitude, the child will not cooperate and the diet will not work. Think of the diet as a gift to your child—a gift of freedom from seizures and the side effects of medication. Don't think of it as a punishment.

Q *Won't my child gain weight on all that fatty food?*

A The amount of food is carefully calculated so that your child will eat all the calories and protein needed for good health, but not so many that weight is gained. The fat content of the food has no bearing on weight as long as overall calories are strictly limited. Although restricting calories is important for achieving seizure control, calories will be adjusted up or down if the dietitian and physician recommend weight gain or loss, or if abnormal weight gain or loss occurs. It is normal for weight gain to accompany growth in height, but even this growth may be slowed while your child is on the diet. Height and weight will catch up when your child returns to a normal diet.

Q *Suppose my daughter eats a piece of toast. Will she go out of ketosis? Will I have to start over?*

A Yes, she may go out of ketosis, but you will not have to start over. You may, however, need to bring your child back into ketosis by skipping a meal or two until ketones in the urine reach the 4+level, then start meals again as usual. If a mistake like this causes a breakthrough seizure, it will not spoil the long-term effects of the diet. Even so, loss of ketosis should be kept to a minimum.

Q *My child was seizure-free on the diet for 3 weeks but had a seizure yesterday. Why?*

A Several potential causes for a breakthrough seizure can occur in a child who has been well controlled on the diet. Eating food that is not part of the meal plans may cause breakthrough seizures. Family members and others often do not understand the need for strict compliance, and they slip food to the child, thinking they are being nice. Older and more mobile children are more likely to break the diet on their own.

Incorrect preparation of foods, or purchasing a new commercial food product not calculated into a meal plan, can also lead to problems. Medications containing glucose or carbohydrates, and even the sucrose in suntan lotion or lipstick may result in seizures.

Illness frequently causes breakthrough seizures in some children. Infections, kidney stones, and severe constipation are other potential causes of breakthrough seizures.

If a breakthrough seizure occurs in a child who has been well controlled on the diet, it is almost always due to an aberration or mistake, and seizure control can easily be reestablished.

Q *If my child has a seizure after being well controlled for 3 weeks on the diet, what should I do?*

A Stay calm. Remember how far your child has come since starting on the diet. Then investigate to see if you can trace—and eliminate—the cause. First, check to see if your child ate something extra. Could a friend have offered a spare cookie? Might Grandma have slipped in a chocolate? Is the dog's food sealed tightly? Is the toothpaste missing? Have any new or different medicines or vitamin supplements been taken? Just a spoonful of regular cough syrup or "sugarless" foods containing sugar substitutes with carbohydrate, such as mannitol, sorbitol, polydextrose, or maltodextrin, can cause breakthrough seizures.

Next, review your preparation methods. Did you do anything different? Did you weigh vegetables raw that should have been cooked? Buy a new brand of sausage? Measuring oil by volume instead of by weight could be a problem if you are using a large amount of oil. All food should be measured on a gram scale.

Is your child gaining weight? Weight gain is one sign that the diet is not being properly calculated or prepared. Seizures may continue or recur if the diet is providing more calories than your child's body needs to maintain itself. In such a case, the calorie count may need to be reduced slightly. Because every child's situation is different, you must do some sleuthing to solve the problem. Your doctor or dietitian may also be able to isolate the possible cause of seizures by listening to you and carefully reviewing your child's diet.

If your child was previously having frequent seizures and then was seizure-free for several weeks on the diet, the diet is likely to be effective despite the breakthrough seizures—it just needs finetuning.

Q *I am doing everything my doctor told me, but my child's seizures are continuing. What more can I do?*

A With your dietician, go over the diet and your home circumstances with a fine-tooth comb to be sure no mistakes are being made in preparation or that anyone is giving unplanned food. Perhaps better seizure control could be achieved with fewer calories. Changing to a more restrictive 4.5:1 ratio of fat to protein plus carbohydrate for a few months may help. In some cases, a 5:1 ketogenic ratio is needed.

Some children on the ketogenic diet will continue to have some seizures. The goal of the diet is to reduce the number and intensity of seizures as much as you can; complete control is not always possible. In the end, it is up to you to decide whether the diet's rigor is worth the level of seizure control and freedom from medications that it provides your child. Some children's seizures do not respond or do not respond sufficiently well to continue the diet.

Q *Is the ketogenic diet nutritionally complete?*

A The ketogenic diet is deficient in multivitamins, trace minerals, and calcium. The ketogenic diet is nutritionally complete only when proper supplements are taken in sugar-free form.

No data shows carnitine is either necessary or useful as a supplement for all children. Because carnitine is expensive, we do not use it unless a child is weak and lacks energy. Then we use it as a test for several weeks. If the child improves, we continue it. Some nutritionists have also claimed that the diet is deficient in trace minerals such as zinc and selenium. All we can say is that we have treated scores of children without any evidence of adverse effects from the absence of micronutrients.

Q *What can my child eat at school?*

A Your dietitian will help you plan meals that can easily be transported to school. Tuna, egg, or chicken salads are particularly easy to carry in sealed plastic containers. Warm or chilled food can be carried in a small cooler or insulated bag, or wrapped in foil. Your child must learn to tell teachers and classmates, "No, thanks!" when snacks are distributed to the class. For occasions such as birthday parties, you can send a container of special cheesecake or frozen eggnog (see Chapter 16) that can be eaten when the other kids eat their cake. It is remarkable how even young children of 4 or 5 years can learn to refuse treats, saying, "I'm a special kid on a special diet."

Q *Can we go to a restaurant or on a day's outing while my child is on the diet?*

A With imagination and planning, you and your child can go anywhere on the diet. On short trips, you can take one or more pre-prepared meals in a cooler. You can ask to have a pre-prepared meal heated in a restaurant's microwave. Ketogenic eggnog or macadamia nuts (sometimes mixed with calculated butter) can serve as occasional easy meal replacements if you are in transit at mealtime.

Q *Can we still go on family trips?*

A You may go on longer trips if all the ingredients of your child's diet are under your control. You can stay in a hotel or motel with a kitchenette, where you can prepare your own or your child's meals. You can order plain grilled chicken, steamed vegetables or fresh fruit, butter, and heavy whipping cream at a restaurant, and weigh portions on your scale when the food arrives. Remember, though, that tiny bits of extra foods such as catsup, dill pickle, or lemon juice can upset your child's ketosis if they are not calculated into the meal. For greater detail on how to preserve your mobility while on the diet, see Chapter 10.

Q *The amounts of food allowed in the diet are so small—won't my child feel hungry?*

A Ketosis suppresses appetite, so children on the diet are not usually as hungry as other children. The diet provides only about three-quarters of the calories that would usually be recommended for a child's height and weight. However, ketosis and the concentration of fat in the diet help to create a full feeling in the stomach despite the small quantity of food. Some children feel hungry for the first week or two of the diet, but their stomachs usually adjust with time. More food may decrease ketosis and actually increase the child's hunger.

Q *What if my child refuses to eat all the food in a meal?*

A All the food in a meal must be consumed at one time—it may not be saved until the next meal or eaten between meals.

There are few things in a child's life that she can control. Eating is one of them. You, the parent, are in a difficult position with the ketogenic diet. You are told that the child must eat everything on her plate. What if she refuses? Give her approximately 20 minutes to eat her meal. If she hasn't eaten, then throw it away and wait for the next meal. If you are placed in the position of coaxing or wheedling your child into eating "just two more bites," you will lose. On occasion, we have seen parents placed in the position where every meal is a battle that extends from one meal to the next. We have even seen a mother finally hire a sitter just to feed the child (in 20 minutes) and break the pattern. The diet goes more smoothly when parents learn to be more relaxed about feeding and children learn that they are not ultimately in control.

Q *My daughter is doing so well on the diet. She has had no seizures. But there is a flu going around, and she vomited all last evening. This afternoon her ketones are low. Why? What should I do?*

A The low ketones may well be due to the infection and the alterations in her metabolism caused by her illness. Because she has been doing so well on the diet, you should probably do nothing. She will most likely be back to eating by morning. In the meantime, you should make sure she gets enough liquid to stay hydrated. If she has stopped vomiting, you might try offering sips of her ketogenic eggnog; because every sip is balanced in terms of its ketogenic ratio, it does not matter if your child only drinks a little bit.

If dehydration becomes a problem, it may be necessary to give some Pedialyte™ (a chemically balanced fluid available at the drugstore). Pedialyte™ contains about 23g of carbohydrate per 1,000cc. When the child is not eating any food, the carbohydrate in Pedialyte™ often is no greater than the combined protein and carbohydrate allotment in the diet, so Pedialyte™ rarely upsets ketosis. In case of severe dehydration, it may be necessary to get an intravenous saline solution at the hospital. Intravenous dextrose should not be used because it will upset ketosis. Another option is CeraLyte™, a solution based on rice, rather than sugar, that can be purchased in stores. We have occasionally used this for our ketogenic diet patients.

Q *What if my daughter has a seizure while she is sick with the flu?*

A Illness often precipitates seizures, even while on the diet. Illness may also sometimes cause a transient drop in ketone levels, and this can precipitate seizures. If your daughter starts to have seizures during an illness, following recovery, you can put her on a fast for one to three meals until she goes back into ketosis and then restart the diet, perhaps at half quantity for a few meals. The effectiveness of the diet is only partly represented by high levels of ketones in the urine. Some children have seizures even while their urinary ketones remain high, while others may do well despite a transient drop in ketones. The most important measure is how well the child is doing.

Q *My son got bronchitis, and his doctor prescribed an antibiotic. How do I know if this will affect the diet?*

A All medicines and pharmaceuticals, from toothpaste to cough syrup, vitamins, and prescription medicine, must, *whenever possible,* be free of all sugar and carbohydrate. Some common forms of sugar and carbohydrate to watch out for on labels are glucose, sucrose, fructose, dextrose, sorbitol, and mannitol. Medication in chewable or tablet form often contains some carbohydrate to bind the tablet together, and sweet-tasting elixirs or syrups often contain sugar. Ask your doctor to prescribe needed medications in sugar-free and carbohydrate-free forms. If you have questions, the best source of information is your pharmacist. In fact, a pharmacist is often an important part of the ketogenic diet team, helping parents through their child's illnesses throughout the duration of the diet by making up sugar-free medications. If your pharmacist cannot help, go directly to the manufacturer. Formulas often change; read labels carefully, and don't take anything for granted.

In an emergency, or if it is not possible to find a sugar-free formula, take care of your child's health first. If losing ketosis is a price that must be paid for your child's health then, after the illness, your child can always fast again and reinstitute the diet. (See Appendix A for more details on medications.)

Q *The ketogenic diet is making my child constipated. How do I keep this from being a problem?*

A Constipation is the most common problem we see in children on the diet, especially during the first week. On the ketogenic diet, smaller amounts of food are eaten, therefore children will have smaller bowel movements or even a BM every other day. This is not necessarily constipation, but may be simply the "nothing in, nothing out" principle. Constipation occurs when the bowel movements are hard, like little balls, and sometimes difficult to pass. Here are a few anti-constipation measures you can try:

- Use meal plans that contain as much fiber as possible. You are allowed to use two lettuce leaves, or about one-half cup of chopped lettuce, per day as a "free" food, and you can use calculated mayonnaise as dressing. Using more Group A vegetables can also help, because you can serve twice as many of these as of Group B vegetables.
- Try cutting out meal plans with catsup, chocolate, or other carbohydrate-based flavorings that take away from the quantity of fiber-rich vegetables your child can eat.

- MiraLax™ powder rarely fails. It is given with water, typically about a tablespoon every day to every other day. It works like a charm.

In extreme cases, you can use a stool softener, such as Colace, or a gentle laxative, such as Milk of Magnesia, diluted Baby Fleet enemas, or other children's rectal suppositories. One mother used a diluted enema regularly every other day, pouring out two-thirds of the dosage so that the long-term use would not hurt her son's bowels. MCT oil, in small amounts, may be calculated into the diet to relieve constipation (see Chapter 14). For more on constipation, see Chapter 9.

Q *Is it possible for my child to become too ketotic?*

A Yes, but rarely. With illness, the level of ketone bodies may become unusually high, and your child may experience shallow, panting breathing. If this happens, give him a sip of orange juice or a cracker to bring the ketone levels back in the normal-high ketone range. If your child becomes both too ketotic and too dehydrated (not taking enough fluid and not passing enough urine), the physician or the hospital may have to give some fluids intravenously. They may, if necessary, give a small amount of glucose. When your child perks up, the diet can be resumed. If excess ketosis becomes a recurring problem, the dietitian can try reducing the child's ketogenic ratio to 3:1.

Q *When should the diet be stopped?*

A Whenever its burdens are greater than its value. For some children, this happens after only a few months. Typically, children who do well on the diet stay on for about 2 years, similar to medicines. However, some children stay on the diet for as long as 6 years or more due to excellent seizure improvement and ease of use. The most common reason to stop the diet during the first year is if it is not working sufficiently well.

Q *The fast during diet initiation sounds terrible. Do I really need to starve my child?*

A Although some evidence suggests that diet initiation can be successful without fasting, we continue to recommend fasting during the initiation phase until ketosis is reached. Fasting gives the child a jump-start into ketosis, and the fast, just by itself, often leads to a dramatic improvement in seizures more quickly than starting the diet without fasting. Most families find that the fast is not so terrible in practice. It is often tougher for the parents than the child. Low blood sugar, vomiting, and sleepiness can occur, but are usually short-lived when they do. Most children either sleep through the fast or are more alert because their seizures improve right away. Many families even use short fasts at home during the diet to boost ketones when a child is sick. This topic is discussed in more detail in Chapter 7.

Q *Should the rest of the family cut carbohydrates too?*

A Although it is absolutely not necessary for the entire family to cut carbohydrates, it often helps a child accept the situation a bit better if others are also making sacrifices. This is especially true for large families. No one would expect the entire school to be on this diet, but many families in which the parents and siblings reduce the amount of cakes, cookies, bread, and pasta in plain sight, create a climate where there is better compliance and less desire to cheat.

SECTION II

THE ABC'S OF THE KETOGENIC DIET

CHAPTER SEVEN

INITIATING THE KETOGENIC DIET: A PROCESS

At Johns Hopkins, initiating the ketogenic diet is a process, not an event. The process begins before a child is accepted into the ketogenic diet program. For patients who have been seen in our pediatric epilepsy clinic, parents are informed about the diet, and its advantages and difficulties for their child are discussed. It is suggested that they read this book and become familiar with the diet before deciding to make the commitment.

Patients who live a distance from us are asked to send the child's EEG reports and other medical records for review by the staff. Parents are also asked to write a statement of expectations describing their child and their (the parents') personal goals for the diet. This statement enables us to better comprehend the parents' goals and expectations. Parents who expect a "cure" are likely to be disappointed. Parents who desire a decrease in their child's seizure frequency or in the medication toxicity are more likely to have their goals achieved.

We have had no firm criteria for accepting or rejecting children for diet initiation at Johns Hopkins. In general, however:

- Most children have more than two seizures per week.
- Most children have tried at least two anticonvulsants without achieving seizure control. Occasionally, we accept children whose seizures have been controlled but only at the expense of medication toxicity.
- Most parents have realistic goals and positive attitudes.

Since children with infantile spasms or Doose syndrome (a syndrome featuring drop seizures), as well as those with the Lennox-Gastaut pattern, may be more likely to respond to the diet than to medication, we are more likely to accept them for the diet earlier in the course of their epilepsy.

> **THE KETOGENIC DIET** should *not* be saved for a last resort only when a child has failed multiple medications. The diet should be considered early in the course of epilepsy, and possibly should be tried after two medications have failed to control the seizures. In some cases, it is used even earlier in the course of epilepsy.

After being scheduled for diet initiation, parents are asked to keep a seizure calendar for the month before hospitalization, to watch the video "Introduction to the Ketogenic Diet," and to read this book. The child's primary care physician is sent information about the diet, along with recommendations for treatment of illness while on the diet. The family's physician must become a member of the ketogenic diet team.

THE ADMISSIONS PROCESS

Just before admission at Johns Hopkins (other centers may have slightly different practices), a child is evaluated as an outpatient, and the parents attend their first lesson on the history of the diet, which includes an overview of the expected course of the hospitalization.

Starting the diet at Hopkins then requires 4 days of hospitalization, beginning with fasting and followed by the gradual introduction of the high-fat meals. During the initial phase of the diet, which lasts several weeks, the body gradually becomes adjusted to the smaller portions and lower calorie levels of the diet as well as to digesting the larger quantities of fat. Several weeks may be required for the individual's body to learn to utilize the fat for energy and for the child's energy level to return to normal. During this period, the family also becomes accustomed to weighing and measuring all meals and to reading food labels, and the child gradually becomes adjusted to the foods of the diet and to not eating other foods.

Debate continues about whether the ketogenic diet must be initiated in the hospital, and about whether it needs to be begun with fasting. The ketogenic diet was originally begun by fasting patients for as long as 25 days, giving only water. In the 1960s, doctors at Johns Hopkins fasted patients until they had lost 10 percent of their body weight, which usually occurred in 10 days. To make the diet more humane, we later developed a protocol using 48 hours of fasting. We have since moved to our current protocol of just 36 hours of fasting. (See Appendix B, "Johns Hopkins Hospital order sheets").

We believe that the initial fast is useful. The fasting jump-starts the ketosis. After 36 hours of fasting, a child is usually in deep ketosis and any food looks good. Gradual introduction of the diet, increasing from one-third of the prescribed amount to two-thirds and then to the full diet, enables the child to adjust to the fatty food and to achieve good ketosis (and often a reduction in seizures) before he goes home.

We introduce the diet with a "keto shake," a milkshake-like meal that is easy to calculate and that may also be frozen into keto ice cream or microwaved into creamy scrambled eggs. We have found that offering one-third of a regular diet meal at initiation is unattractive: It comes to a sprig of broccoli on one edge of a large plate, a thumbnail-sized piece of turkey on another, and a swallow of cream. The parent's usual reaction is "Arrrgh!!" Initiating the diet with a "keto shake" avoids this unpleasant experience and also eliminates mistakes by our hospital's dietary service.

PROBLEMS WITH DIET INITIATION

When the protocol described above is followed, we have occasionally seen children become too ketotic and begin vomiting. Reversal of this condition requires some orange juice (about 30cc) and a small amount of sugar to restore balance. We have on rare occasions seen children develop symptomatic hypoglycemia, which is heralded by a decreased responsiveness and sometimes pallor and sweating. Hypoglycemia is also responsive to a small amount of orange juice with sugar. These unusual but potentially serious side effects are part of why we prefer to have children in the hospital during the diet initiation, where they can be closely observed and treated if necessary. We consider these side effects to be bumps along the road and not complications of the diet.

Sometimes the problems at initiation are psychological. We are leery of making a mother deny food to her child for this prolonged period of time without the support of the medical staff and of other mothers. Not feeding your child is a very unnatural and difficult thing to do.

We also find that the 4-day hospital stay gives parents the opportunity to focus on the diet, to learn how to calculate meals, and to learn the purpose for what they will be doing. We feel that the intense (2 hours per day) instructional process is a key element in our success.

Have we tested each of these elements? No. Are they all necessary? We don't know. Can the diet be initiated without fasting? This has been done at other centers, and apparently can be effective. Can the diet be initiated without hospitalization? This, too, has been done.

However, at Hopkins we continue with the protocol that has brought our patients such success: 4 days of hospitalization with 2 hours of teaching each day.

On the fourth day after hospital admission, the child is discharged home with three "keto shakes" for the journey. This marks the end of the initiation process and the beginning of the "fine-tuning" phase.

FINE-TUNING THE DIET

Fine-tuning the ketogenic diet begins after discharge and is usually done by phone. It involves the dietitians adjusting the various components of the diet—calories, liquids, fats, recipes, ketogenic ratios, and so forth—to achieve the best level of ketosis for optimal seizure control. Fine-tuning is a critical part of achieving success on the diet and is discussed further in Chapter 8.

GETTING READY FOR THE DIET: THE PARENTS' PERSPECTIVE

Psychological preparation

The most important factor contributing to the success of the ketogenic diet is the family's psychological state. Committing to the diet requires a great deal of faith. The parents must believe that the diet can work. It requires determination to get a child out of that medication haze; to stop those frustrating absence seizures; to throw away the helmet that had to be worn as protection against head-drop seizures.

Parents who start out as doubters will focus on the inevitable initial difficulties of the diet instead of focusing on the decrease in seizures and the improved behavior of the child as the diet starts. Without faith, it will be too frustrating when the child accidentally uses the wrong toothpaste, when she is irritable and demanding, or when she gets sick and has a seizure 3 weeks into the treatment. It will be too sad for these parents to bear if the child cries for afternoon cookies or Sunday night pizza.

If parents start out thinking positively, saying, "We will do whatever is necessary to give this diet a chance to work, the sacrifice is worthwhile if our child has a chance to become seizure-free," then they are already halfway there. Most children have fewer seizures and/or require less medicine on the diet. The question then becomes whether the improvement is sufficient to continue the diet. Families have a greater chance of success if they think of the opportunity to try the diet as a gift to the child, not as a punishment for having seizures.

Sometimes problems with the diet may not come from the parents or the child. They may come from a

"How-will-my-grandchild-know-it's-me-if-I-don't-bring- Hershey's-Kisses?" grandma, or from a jealous "How-come-Peter-gets-all-the-attention?" sister. The optimism and faith that will carry a family through the diet (pardon us if this sounds a bit preachy) has to come from a team effort, encompassing the whole family, especially the child. Once the diet is effective and the seizures are under better control, once the child is functioning better, it becomes much easier to maintain the momentum. At the start, it can be very tough. It is the willingness of the parents to meet the challenge that will carry the family through.

AT FIRST YOU ARE GOING TO BE AFRAID *of temptation. You're going to feel bad about your child seeing others eat food he can't have. You'll be worried about what the diet's emotional effects will be. And you're going to be worried about whether your kid will cooperate. But you can live through it!*

If you have other kids, they can eat other foods. Try to be positive.

The main thing to remember is, if the diet works, your kid will be so happy to feel well again!

—CC

I REALLY HAVE TO THANK YOU SO MUCH *for putting me on the ketogenic diet back in 1991. I know that before I went on the ketogenic diet to help my seizures, I was on a lot of medication. The medication really did not help my seizures and made me have behavior and learning problems. If it was not for you, I don't think I would have made it this far in life. I am not sick anymore with seizures, and I can concentrate and focus on my schoolwork. I am in college, sleeping away during the week, and doing great. I am so grateful to have had you as my doctor. Once again, thank you so much.*

—AC

STATEMENT OF EXPECTATIONS

At Johns Hopkins, we ask that each parent write a statement of expectations, including a definition of what "success" on the diet would mean, and send it to us before the hospital admission.

Some parents write that success would be if the child's seizures were reduced by half, others demand complete seizure control. Some say, "If we could only decrease or eliminate the medication, then we could see what she is really like. We can live with the seizures, it is the medication which is so difficult."

These statements force parents to confront the question of what they expect of the diet. The statements also frequently offer substantial insight into a parent's strengths, desires, and ability to confront reality. The written statement can create an opportunity for a physician to discuss misunderstandings about the diet or misperceptions about a child's potential abilities. Parents often hope that the child's problems are all due to the medications, or only due to the seizures, and that the diet will miraculously make their child like one who was never ill.

The written statement of expectations clarifies their beliefs. Filed in the child's medical chart, the statement also offers a benchmark against which to assess progress when the child returns for follow-up. At the follow-up visit we often hear, "...but he is still having several drops each week." A reminder that he used to have 50 a day and that he has made substantial progress with decreasing medications can be helpful in keeping the child on the diet. A reminder of what the parents wrote: "If only the seizures decreased by half," "If only we could get rid of some of the medication," "If only she wasn't so tired all of the time," is frequently very helpful in reminding the family just how far they've come.

GETTING THE CHILD'S COOPERATION

The diet is more likely to go more smoothly if children are enlisted—rather than ordered—to participate. Children do not like having seizures. They do not like being different from their friends. Often, the thing they hate most is taking medications. They want to be cured of their seizures. If possible, explain to a child, in an age-appropriate fashion, how the diet may help fix these problems. If parents communicate their own enthusiasm for the diet as something worth trying, something that really might work, most children will buy in. They will feed on your enthusiasm. So don't start the diet if you and your child are not enthusiastic about trying it—without that enthusiasm, it will be too hard.

But no one should make promises that cannot be kept! Parents cannot guarantee to the child that the seizures will disappear completely or that there will be no more medication. These are goals, but they cannot be promises.

Sticking to the diet is ultimately the child's responsibility. Parents can help by giving children the psychological and emotional power to handle the tough parts. Role-playing may be useful. Parents can try rehearsing what to say in difficult situations. For example, a parent might pretend to be a teacher offering a cracker at snack time, to let a child practice saying, "That's not on my diet, thank you!" Or, a parent might pretend to be a friend trying to swap a sandwich for the child's cheesecake at lunch, to teach the child responses such as, "No, I'm on a magic diet. I have to eat my own food." Children on the diet usually exhibit amazing self-control and willpower. They often handle the diet far better than their parents do—especially when they are doing well.

An example is Sarah, who had a stroke at birth and was 5 years old when she first came to Hopkins. Her one-sided seizures were hard to control, and she was a candidate for surgery. But before undergoing brain surgery, her family decided to try the ketogenic diet. Sarah did very well, and her seizures were better for a time, but ultimately she did not have good enough seizure control. Surgery was scheduled. Sarah would say, "What I dream about is having French fries again when I'm not on the diet any more." So, the night before surgery a nurse brought Sarah French fries. Sarah's response was "I can't have these. I'm still on my special diet."

Older children who try the ketogenic diet often need someone on whom they can vent their anger and frustrations. It is far better if this can be someone other than his parents. For teens and preteens, it may help to set up special telephone times when they can call and talk to someone, perhaps a counselor or a mentor who has already been through the diet. This may start with a weekly call and then gradually become less frequent. Through these calls, children can report successes and discuss problems, receive reinforcement, and hear stories about others who went through the same thing.

One of our counselor's favorite lines, when things seem particularly bleak and a child wants to quit the diet, is "Hey, it's up to you. No one is making you stay on the diet. You are always free to choose to stop the diet, to go back to having seizures and taking medicine. It's all up to you." Giving the responsibility to the child eliminates the parents and counselor as bad guys, and empowers the child to see the reality that, if the diet is indeed working, the choices are really very simple.

WHEN MICHAEL BEGAN TO MOAN FOR A COOKIE, *I told him, "Michael, the epilepsy is your problem, and you have to solve it. We are here to help you, but most of the work is going to be yours. You're a big guy, you can handle it.*

—EH

(Update: Michael stuck with the diet and now has been off it for several years. He still has a rare seizure, but does well in school and is a firstrate basketball player.)

SPECIAL EQUIPMENT

The essential pieces of equipment for the ketogenic diet are a gram scale and a kit to test ketones in the urine. The rest of the items listed in this section are things that other parents have found helpful.

Gram scales

The gram scale is the main calculating tool for the diet, so it is extremely important. Parents must either buy a gram scale or make sure that the hospital plans to supply one for the family to take home. At Johns Hopkins, we make a gram scale available to parents at cost. Providing this service ensures that all parents get an accurate scale while saving them the time and effort of searching for one themselves. The scale should be accurate, should display weights in one-tenth gram increments, and should be portable.

Scales can be obtained through office-supply or kitchen-supply stores. Electronic digital scales, although slightly more expensive, are more accurate to the gram than manual scales. Examples of suitable scales include the Pelouse electronic postal scale and the Ohaus portable electronic postal scale.

Testing for urinary ketones

Strips for testing ketone levels in the urine are commonly available in drugstores, often combined with the glucose tests used by diabetic patients (made by Bayer™ and available over the counter). Keto-Diastix, manufactured by the Ames Company, is one such test strip. Children on the ketogenic diet test urine daily with these "Ketostix."

Testing for blood in the urine

Parents are instructed to test the urine weekly for blood, which may be an early sign of kidney stones, one of the fairly common side effects of the diet. Hemoglobin (blood) in the urine may be tested using Bayer' Multistix 10SG, which tests for several things, including hemoglobin and ketones.

Because these strips are expensive, we recommend using them only once each week. A positive test for hemoglobin does *not* necessarily mean blood is present in the urine. The test should be repeated on several different specimens and then confirmed by a physician before a parent should become concerned.

Optional equipment that may be useful

Parents have found a variety of equipment helpful while their children are on the ketogenic diet. The following is a list gathered from many parents. It is meant as a source of ideas. All this equipment is optional. Parents may buy these supplies if and as needed:

- Large collection of small plastic storage containers
- Bendable straws for drinking every drop
- Sippy cups for smaller children
- Screw-top plastic beverage containers
- Small rubber spatulas to be used as plate-cleaners

- One-, two-, four-, and six-ounce plastic cups
- Measuring cup marked with milliliters or a graduated cylinder for weighing and measuring
- 10cc syringe
- Pyrex custard dishes for microwave cooking and freezing meals
- Popsicle molds
- Six-inch nonstick skillet for sautéing individual portions and easy clean-up
- Travel cooler and/or insulated bag (useful to take home keto shake from hospital)
- One or two small Thermos jugs for school and travel
- Toothpicks for picking up morsels of food to make eating fun
- Blender
- Milkshake wand or small hand beater
- Portable dual-burner electric camping stove for trips
- Masking tape for labels
- Microwave oven

To repeat, it is not necessary to own a lot of equipment before starting the diet. The above is simply a sample list from various parents. Parents will gain more insight as to what equipment they will need, as well as specific brands of food that are acceptable, during their in-hospital ketogenic diet education. The only supplies that are absolutely necessary before starting the diet are a scale that measures in grams (to weigh foods) and strips for testing ketone levels in urine, which may be purchased or obtained from the hospital.

SPECIAL FOODS

Heavy whipping cream

THE ONLY ESSENTIAL FOOD RESEARCH parents must do before starting the diet is to find out whether their neighborhood heavy whipping cream supply is 36 percent fat, 40 percent fat, or somewhere in-between. The fat content of heavy whipping cream varies from one location to another, but most heavy cream is 36 percent fat.

The fat content of available cream affects the calculation of the diet, so it is important to find what is available in a given neighborhood and to tell the dietitian before the child's diet is calculated. Make sure that no sugar is added!

If you have any doubts about the fat content of your local cream, call the dairy directly. Dairies are required by law to know the fat percentage of the cream they supply. Remember: Labeling laws do not require companies to list anything less than 1g of carbohydrate, protein, or fat, although fractional grams can affect the ketogenic diet! Once you find an acceptable brand, stick with it. Some local dairies will help to ensure that your local store stocks large containers of heavy whipping cream. Call your local dairy if you have any questions.

Flavorings

Many parents use flavorings to make the diet more fun for kids. These include:

- Baking chocolate (must be calculated into the child's diet)

- Fruit-flavored sugar-free, caffeine-free diet soda such as Faygo or Wal-Mart Free & Clear
- Pure flavoring extracts: vanilla, almond, lemon, maple, coconut, chocolate. Make certain that they are pure, and check for alcohol content. Pure flavorings may be ordered from Bickford Flavorings (216-531-6006, or 1-800-283-8322)
- Sugar-free flavored gelatin such as D-Zerta, Jell-O, or Royal
- Non-stick spray such as Pam or Mazola No-stick for cooking
- Carbohydrate-free, calorie-free, sweeteners. Saccharin (1/4grain tablets of pure saccharin) is best. Splenda and Stevia are also OK, but liquid versions of these are always best. Other sweeteners, such as Equal (the blue packets), Sweet 'n' Low (the pink packets), and NutraSweet contain carbohydrates that can upset ketosis. The liquid form of these is preferred.

This list, like the equipment list, is intended as a source of ideas, not a must-buy-right-away order. The rest of the diet ingredients should be pure, fresh, simple foods: lean meat, fish, or poultry, bacon, eggs, cheese, fruit, vegetables, butter, mayonnaise, and canola or olive oil.

READ THE LABEL! When using processed foods, be sure to read the label carefully at all times. Manufacturers often change the formulations of their products without prior notice. Therefore, each time you buy a processed food product, even if you have used it before, you must read the label very carefully. Remember that labeling laws do not require disclosure of contents less than 1g. Call the manufacturer if you have any questions.

Beware of hidden carbohydrates

Pay close attention to any foods or medicines that may contain carbohydrates. Nonsugar carbohydrates include mannitol, sorbitol, dextrin, and many ingredients ending in "-ose," such as maltose, lactose, fructose, glucose, sucrose, dextrose, or polycose. All these are carbohydrates and can be broken down into glucose. They either should not be used or must be calculated into the diet. Many foods, candies, and gums that are billed as "sugar-free" are not carbohydrate-free and cannot be used on the ketogenic diet.

BARBARA HAD HAD NO SEIZURES *in 6 months and was doing superbly well on the ketogenic diet. In preparation for her follow-up EEG, the technician inadvertently gave her liquid chloral hydrate to allow her to sleep. But the oral chloral hydrate was in a carbohydrate base. The technician should have used carbohydrate-free chloral hydrate suppositories instead. It does not take much carbohydrate to quickly negate ketosis. Barbara's first seizure in 6 months occurred during that EEG.*

MICHELLE LIVED IN THE CITY BUT, *during the summer, the family spent weekends at their beach house. She did well on the diet throughout the winter, with a marked decrease in seizure* frequency. In the summer, she again began having increased seizures, although only on weekends. The family would go to their summer house on Fridays. By Saturday, Michelle's ketones would be low, and her seizures would increase. Her parents turned themselves inside out attempting to find the reason. They checked the foods, the environment, and finally decided she must be allergic to the beach and their pool. They were about to sell the house.

At last, together with a nurse from Johns Hopkins, they again went over everything they did on Friday and Saturday. "When we arrived at the beach, we lathered Michelle with suntan lotion," they told the nurse. Aha! They checked the suntan lotion label: It was in a sorbitol base. Apparently, enough sorbitol was absorbed through Michelle's skin to affect her ketones and alter her seizure threshold! After switching to a sorbitolfree suntan lotion, the family continued *taking Michelle to the beach with no recurrence of seizures.*

Teenagers on the diet have reported that some lipsticks and soaps containing sorbitol may lead to seizures. Lowering ketosis through consumption of carbohydrates does not always cause breakthrough seizures, but it can. The good news is that when isolated breakthrough seizures occur, they nearly always can be eliminated again once the source is traced.

Medications

Medications play an important role in the ultimate success of the ketogenic diet. Starches and sugars are frequently used as fillers and taste enhancers in all forms of medication—tablets, capsules, and particularly liquid medications. These starches and sugars can easily be overlooked in diet formulation, but they can impair a child's ability to maintain high levels of ketosis. Read the labels of all medications carefully. Take into account the carbohydrate content of all medications, whether routine medications taken daily or intermittent medications given to treat conditions such as a cold or an infection.

Ideally, the total carbohydrate content in medications should be less than 0.g (or 100mg) for the entire day. Anything higher should be calculated into the meal plan's daily carbohydrate allotment. For example, a child taking 0.09g (90mg) of phenobarbital at bedtime in the form of three 0.03g (30mg) tablets receives 0.07g (72mg) of starch and lactose per tablet, or a daily total of 0.21g (216mg). Carbohydrate-free forms of most of the older anticonvulsants are available. For example, valproate and topiramate in the sugar-free form of sprinkles can be used. Some of the new anticonvulsants do not come in sugar-free or carbohydrate-free form. If they must be continued, the carbohydrate content should be calculated into the diet. In some instances, the sugar-free intravenous form of the medication can be used orally. During the fasting and dietinitiation phase of the diet, the carbohydrate content of medications should be minimized by avoiding liquid preparations. The filler in pills may be ignored or calculated into the carbohydrates allotted. Pills can always be crushed and given in heavy whipping cream, ketogenic eggnog, or even unsweetened yogurt.

Difficulty in prescribing medications for a child on the ketogenic diet often arises from the fact that many common over-the-counter and prescription medications are not available in a sugar-free form. Many of those listed as "sugar-free" in references are appropriate for use in the diabetic population, but not for children on the ketogenic diet because they contain starch or carbohydrates in the form of sugar substitutes such as sorbitol and mannitol.

THE FOOD AND DRUG ADMINISTRATION (FDA) does not require the listing of inactive ingredients, such as sorbitol, in the labeling of oral prescription drugs. Even when ingredients are listed, their precise amounts are not often found on the label.

Manufacturers are also frequently reluctant to release information about the amounts of particular ingredients in a medication, contending that this is proprietary information or that formulations change frequently. However, they can usually be persuaded to release the information if it is for treatment of a specific patient.

A pharmacist who is willing to get to know the ketogenic diet and the child, and to work with the family for the duration of the diet, can be a valuable asset, helping to interpret labels and calling manufacturers if necessary. When starting the diet, locate a source of sugar-free, carbohydrate-free, and lactose-free multivitamins, toothpaste, and calcium supplements. Ask your pharmacist or dietitian to double-check the contents of specific brands, because formulas can change:

- Multivitamins: Mead Johnson's Poly-Vi-Sol (liquid or drops) with iron or Mead Johnson's Unicap-M
- Carbohydrate-free calcium: Rugby's calcium gluconate (600 to 650mg) or Calci-Mix (500mg)

- Carbohydrate-free toothpaste: Tom's Natural, Arm & Hammer, Ultra Bright

Routine medications that are taken daily should come from a single company, because ingredient concentrations vary among manufacturers. General rules for the use of medications, a selected list of medications that have been used by children on the diet, and contact information for pharmaceutical manufacturers can be found in Appendix A of this book. Most medications can also be made in a carbohydrate-free form by a compounding pharmacy. You can ask a local pharmacy to do this, or order from H&B Pharmacy (201-997-2010).

GETTING READY FOR THE DIET: THE KETOGENIC DIET TEAM

A team effort is needed to keep each child and family on track and help them to get through the challenges of the initiation and fine-tuning period. The ketogenic diet team, or "ketoteam," at Hopkins includes a physician, dietitian, nurse, and counselor who are all familiar with the diet. Each plays an important role in both initiating and maintaining the diet.

The size of the team will depend on the institution and its ketogenic diet program. The dietitian must allocate enough time not only to teach the diet while the family is in the hospital for diet initiation, but also to help the family with questions and dietary changes after discharge. Some medical centers also have a nurse or physician's assistant who can help the family through the many small crises that do not require medical attention.

If a center is going to start children on the diet, it must also be prepared to adjust the diet and work with the family through the fine-tuning period for at least several months after discharge. We estimate that an average family requires 40 telephone hours of dietary and illness counseling during the first year on the diet. The child and family are, of course, essential partners in the ketoteam as well.

ADMISSION FOR THE START OF THE DIET

At Johns Hopkins, we find that it is easier to admit three or four patients simultaneously for initiation of the ketogenic diet than to do it one at a time. The advantage of admitting several patients at once is not only the efficiency of teaching the daily classes to multiple individuals, but also the support that families in the group can provide to each other as they go through the learning curve and the tribulations of diet initiation together. Without the group, a tendency exists for each parent to feel that he is the only person in the whole world who is burdened with such an overwhelming task. Families in each group often stay in contact after hospital discharge and are brought back to clinic for follow-up on the same day.

Groups are usually admitted every 2 to 4 weeks, which allows us to get one group off to a good start before the next one comes in.

The inpatient hospital stay is 4 days, with an outpatient visit and a teaching session on the day before admission. People often ask why a child has to be hospitalized while starting the diet. The reasons are that in a hospital:

- Physicians can supervise the fasting and guard against potentially serious symptoms of hypoglycemia, dehydration, or severe acidosis.
- Physicians can, if necessary, adjust medication levels according to the child's needs. Although medication should not be reduced more than necessary for several weeks, until the child and family adjust to the diet, it often is necessary to eliminate or sharply reduce phenobarbital and acetazolamide (Diamox) to prevent toxicity and too much sleepiness during the fasting and early acidosis.
- The ketoteam can meet intensively with parents and train them to prepare the diet and deal with common physical and psychosocial issues that may arise.
- Excess ketoacidosis occurs uncommonly when starting the diet,

but may occasionally require either IV fluids (sugarfree) or fluids given by a nasogastric tube.

An example of excess ketoacidosis was Robert, a frail 3-year-old with very difficult-to-control drop spells. His mother was eager to get started on the diet, so she eliminated all starches and carbohydrates three days before coming to Hopkins.

The fasting was started, and the next morning Robert was admitted to the hospital. That night, he vomited once and did not want to take his fluids. The next morning, he was very sleepy. By that evening, he had vomited twice and vomited his first keto shake.

Blood tests showed that Robert was too ketotic and, without enough fluids, he was also somewhat dehydrated. Some fluids and a small amount of glucose put him back on track and allowed him to take the keto shake and progress to the diet.

At one time, we at Hopkins admitted a few children who had tried the diet elsewhere and had shown some promise that the diet was working. Parents would ask if we could make their child completely seizure free. We found that our success rate with these children was similar to those that we initially started on the diet. The dietitians had sometimes miscalculated the number of calories or not made clear to the parents the amount of carbohydrates allowed. Many reasons existed for less-thanoptimal results. However, we no longer admit children whose diet had been initiated elsewhere, because we would be inundated by those who had failed the diet elsewhere.

CHAPTER EIGHT

FINE-TUNING THE DIET: THE KEY TO SUCCESS

Fine-tuning the ketogenic diet involves an adjustment of a child's calories and ketogenic ratio, meal plans, eating patterns, liquid allotments, and other variables in order to achieve optimal seizure control. The first few weeks after a child's discharge from the hospital are often the most intensive fine-tuning period. This initial period of fine-tuning is, we believe, the key to long-term success or failure on the ketogenic diet. Fine-tuning the diet begins after discharge and is usually done by phone or e-mail.

We encourage close communication with the ketoteam as the dietitian adjusts the various components of the diet—calories, liquids, fats, recipes, ketogenic ratios, and so forth—to achieve the best level of ketosis for optimal seizure control and the best meals for the child and the family. This support can be crucial as the family searches for the proper foods, learns to read and interpret labels, becomes accustomed to preparing the diet, and integrates it into their lifestyle. Myriad questions arise as a child's body becomes accustomed to the diet and as the meals are prepared. Support for fine-tuning is particularly necessary when seizure control improves initially but the family is hoping for even better seizure control or for the child to be on even less medication.

Initiating the diet means not only changing the foods that are consumed but also changing the parents' and family members' attitudes and expectations about food and mealtimes. This is particularly true for small children, in whom the small number of calories calculated is overestimated at the start or just seems "too small" and is raised by the parent who cooks, with resultant weight gain for the child and lack of optimal seizure control. A reduction of as little as 10 calories per meal in small children (50 calories per meal in a 6-year-old), may be sufficient to bring about stable weight for the child and better seizure control.

Sometimes a child refuses to eat the cream or becomes too constipated. Adjustments to the child's diet must then be made. It takes at least 2 weeks to see if a change is effective. Since only one change can be made at a time, it may take several months of fine-tuning to see how much benefit the diet will provide for that child.

The fine-tuning phase is often the most time-consuming for the dietitian as the family develops confidence in the diet and the ability to make decisions for themselves. This fine-tuning, and the parental support provided by our experienced dietitians, may be why such a large proportion of families who start the diet at Johns Hopkins stick with the diet, and why smaller programs may be less successful.

The goals of fine-tuning are:
- To reduce seizures to a minimum—optimally for a child to become free of seizures.
- To reduce seizure medications to a minimum—eventually and optimally

for a child to become free of anticonvulsant medications.

Each family is asked to make a 3-month commitment to attempting the diet, in order to give a chance to the fine-tuning phase. We ask this even before the family comes into the hospital to initiate the fasting phase of the diet. Eighty-three percent of our families remain on the diet for at least 3 months. Every family is told that they may discontinue the diet any time they wish, after the 3-month trial. However, because the initiation of the diet is so very labor-intensive for both the family and the ketogenic diet team, this investment of time, effort, and money is not worthwhile for anyone concerned if the diet is not given a good trial.

EXPECTATIONS

Fine-tuning does not always lead to total freedom from seizures. During the initiation of the ketogenic diet and afterward, it helps if a family's expectations are realistic, so that they are not setting themselves up for disappointment. Virtually all families have watched the videotape from the Charlie Foundation before diet initiation. In this tape, it appears that Charlie Abrahams came to Hopkins severely impaired by his seizures and medications and walked out of the hospital 4 days later, cured. This impression is reinforced by the story of the child with uncontrollable seizures in the Meryl Streep film *First Do No Harm.* That child was also flown to Johns Hopkins and sent home cured.

These stories are both *based* on truth, but they are not typical, and certainly not universal.

- Not everyone is cured by the ketogenic diet.
- Not all of those whose seizures are substantially helped by the diet find the correct calorie level and ketogenic ratio during their initial stay in the hospital.
- Not all children are able to come off medication and remain seizure-free.

With careful fine-tuning, however, more than one-half of the children starting the ketogenic diet at Hopkins derive sufficient benefit that they remain on the diet for more than 1 year.

Even Charlie Abrahams required a fine-tuning period. Charlie didn't go home from the hospital in 4 days. He remained several extra days in the hospital, sick and vomiting, until it was determined that a virus was causing his nausea. Even after he had returned home, it took days for Charlie to feel well. After this initial difficult period, Charlie became seizure-free and eventually medication-free. Still, he was often reluctant to eat, and persuading him to finish each meal was a major daily struggle for his mother. Two years later, when coming off the diet, he again had several seizures and had to go back on a modified diet. Eventually, Charlie was able to come off the diet and off medications—and remain seizure free for years.

The lessons to be learned from Charlie's case are important. Charlie's experience with the diet was, and is, a spectacular success. But this success did not come easily. When obstacles arose, his parents refused to become disappointed and discouraged. They put in a lot of hard work, maintained a tough attitude, and made the diet work for Charlie.

The most important thing for a parent to remember during the finetuning period is: You can, and you must, persevere! If your child is doing well at the start of the diet, terrific! But most children do not immediately become seizure-free. Many never become totally free of seizures; others do become virtually, or even totally, seizure-free after weeks or months of careful fine-tuning. Only after working carefully with the ketoteam for several months will you have enough information to decide if your child is experiencing sufficient improvement to continue with the diet.

If seizures are controlled for even a few days at the start, the diet is likely to work. Long-term control can likely be established with patient fine-tuning. We suspect that at the end of 2 days of fasting and the 2 days of gradual introduction of the ketogenic eggnog, a child's blood serum ketones may reach a peak, providing a temporarily high level of seizure control. Once a child is at home and eating meals again, serum ketones may not be as high, even though the urine is still 4+. Increasing the ketosis by fine-tuning the diet may help.

Breakthrough seizures do not necessarily mean that the diet has failed; further fine-tuning is likely to be beneficial. If seizures are improved, less frequent, or less severe, it may be hoped that further improvement can be achieved as the diet is adjusted.

Some factors that may have to be adjusted during this fine-tuning period are calorie allotment and distribution, the ketogenic ratio, meal plans, meal frequency, liquid intake, fiber content, and anticonvulsant medication levels.

THE IMPORTANCE OF SLEUTHING

To master the fine-tuning process, parents and the ketoteam become adept at tracing the cause of any problem that arises. If a child is having problems on the diet, the parents and the rest of the diet team must become private eyes. It often takes a detective's spirit to locate the source of a problem and fix it. The most common cause of a problem with the diet is that the child is getting the wrong amount or the wrong balance of food and liquid. There could be many reasons why the amount or balance of food and liquid are off:

- Is there an opportunity for the child to eat extra food at school or while playing at a friend's house?
- Is the diet prescription correctly calculated? The caloric needs of a disabled child may be much lower than those of a nonhandicapped child of the same age and size.
- Are commercial foods being used? They often contain hidden carbohydrates.
- If commercial foods are used, are they the exact brands and items called for in the menu? For example, different brands of bologna may have different fillers and different carbohydrate contents.
- Check the label—has the manufacturer changed ingredients?
- If calculations were made by computer, are the database entries for the ingredients correct?

- Is the child gaining weight? If so, she is getting too many calories, and the diet must be re-calculated.
- Is the child sick with a common virus or bacterial infection? Infections may trigger seizures both in children on the diet and in those on medications. Wait until the infection is gone, then reassess how the child is doing.
- Is everything being measured on a gram scale except free fluids? Sometimes, after the diet seems to be working well, parents become lax and measure foods "by eye" rather than by scale.
- Are Group B vegetables being measured properly, and differently, from Group A vegetables?
- Are vegetables being weighed cooked or raw, as specified?
- Are canned fruits packed in water, as they should be, rather than in glucose-containing syrup or fruit juice?
- Is a soft-hearted grandparent in the picture encouraging the child to cheat "just a little?"

It is not possible to list every problem and solution in this book, but the principle to remember is: Be a sleuth. Think it through. Don't give up. Look for clues. Was there a change in the number or kind of seizures at a certain time of the day or week? Did the problems begin following a certain meal plan or a specific family event?

JESSICA CAME IN FOR A CHECK-UP *after a year on the diet, and she was doing great. She talked like a little adult, whereas before the diet she had difficulty making sentences at all because her mind was so full of medication and seizures. She was still having some seizures, though. What she told us was that her grandmother liked to give her candy, even though the candy gave her seizures. She said she was going to change that, though. She was going to start saying, "I can't have any more candy, Grandma. I'm on a special diet, and I have to stay on my diet because I don't like having seizures!" Jessica had to stay on the diet for longer than the usual*

*period of time. She would probably
have gotten off sooner if her
grandmother hadn't cheated.*

—MK

If a problem develops after good seizure control has been established, parents should examine every aspect of their child's food and liquid intake, play habits, pharmaceuticals, and time with baby-sitters and relatives. The dietitian should listen to a parent describe exactly how each meal is prepared. If the dietitian cannot solve the problem, the physician may need to get involved. With persistence, you can most likely isolate the problem and correct it.

REMEMBER: Illness, ear infection, the flu, or urinary tract infection may cause breakthrough seizures. See if a child is sick and if the cause of breakthrough seizures might be temporary illness before changing the diet. Illness is the most common cause of breakthrough seizures.

MEASURING KETOSIS

The efficacy of fine-tuning is measured by a child's seizure control, but also by her level of ketosis. It is presumed, although not scientifically proven, that the ketogenic diet produces seizure control by changing the brain's metabolism to one based on ketones rather than carbohydrate. This is achieved by dramatically reducing the child's carbohydrate intake and instead eating a diet high in fat. The incompletely metabolized fat leaves residual ketone bodies, which the brain then uses as its energy source (see Chapter 2). The specific goal of fine-tuning, then, is to get the brain into a state of ketosis adequate to obtain optimal seizure control.

We teach parents to check ketones daily by using a urine dipstick. This is an easy, cost-effective method for monitoring the level of ketosis. The paper stick, when dipped in the child's urine, turns color depending on the amount of ketones in the urine. The ketogenic diet has traditionally been fine-tuned to maintain the child's urine at 3+ to 4+ketones, which turn the stick a dark purple in color (80 to 160mmol).

For babies and young children who are not yet toilet-trained, urine is collected by placing cotton balls in the diaper. Once the child has urinated, the cotton balls can be squeezed onto a dipstick for testing. For older children on the diet, peeing on a dipstick becomes second nature. For older children who are not continent, you can use the cotton ball approach or periodically use a urine-collection bag, available in physician offices.

The weakness of urinary ketone testing is that it is actually the level of ketones in the brain, not those in the urine, that influences seizure control. Ketones in the urine can seem lower if tested after a child drinks a large quantity of liquid. They may vary with the time of day. These ups and downs, however, may have only an indirect relation to seizure control.

We predict that one day, when the instruments are improved to the accuracy of those measuring glucose in diabetics, measuring ketones in the blood may provide a more accurate picture of ketosis relevant to seizure control. Technology is now in development that will allow the measurement of ketones in the blood on a finger-prick of blood, just as diabetics currently measure their own blood sugar. When blood (serum) ketone tests at home are commercially available, the goal of "fine-tuning" the diet may become to produce certain levels of blood ketones, rather than testing the amount that spills out in the urine. However, until serum ketone tests are readily and inexpensively available, urinary assessment remains the best (and only) available tool to monitor a child's ketosis.

Preliminary evidence using blood ketones suggests that once the blood ketone level rises to more than 2mmol, the urine ketone level becomes 4+. That is the highest level the dipsticks can measure. Seizure control however, appears far better when serum levels are greater than 4mmol, way beyond that 4+urine level. So, a urine ketone test of 4+is necessary to establish that the child has ketosis but not sufficient to indicate very good ketosis. It is to be hoped that serum ketone tests may permit a level of seizure control beyond what is now possible.

COMMON PROBLEMS AT THE START OF THE DIET

After the first 2 to 3 weeks following the hospital discharge, the child and the family will have had the chance to adapt to the diet as it was initially calculated. This is the time we start making the small changes we call fine-tuning, which can often make a major difference in a child's level of seizure control. The most common areas to be explored for finetuning potential are:

- Caloric intake
- Carbohydrate intake
- Distribution of meals
- Misuse of free foods
- Menu preparation
- Illness
- Ketogenic ratio
- Fluid intake
- Processed food content
- Function or use of gram scales

- Food values used in calculations

Nearly every child whose seizures are somewhat, but not entirely, controlled on the diet by 2 to 3 weeks after discharge will benefit, to some degree, from a period of fine-tuning.

If indications suggest that a child is being helped by the diet but some problems remain, get into a fine-tuning mode. Be a sleuth. Parents, physicians, and dietitians must work together. Figure out the possible causes of the problems and root them out. Many children of intrepid, optimistic parents continue to improve over the entire course of the first year on the ketogenic diet.

FINE-TUNING MEAL PLANS

As mentioned in Chapter 7, each child is given several (about six) meal plans, calculated by the dietitian specifically for that child, before leaving the hospital at diet initiation. These meal plans will probably be in the form of "chicken (or meat, or egg), Group B vegetable (or 10 percent fruit), fat, cream." As the child adjusts to the diet, the meal plans themselves may need fine-tuning. Physical reasons, such as weight loss or weight gain, may necessitate revising the meal plans, or a child may refuse to eat a basic diet component, such as cream.

As parents prepare the diet meal, they will learn from their child what works and what does not work for them. One child who loves chocolate cream popsicles, for example, may want to eat chocolate cream popsicles at every lunch and dinner. Another child who leaves the hospital with six basic meal plans may grow tired of them after a period and want more variety.

Once parents get the hang of using their gram scales and making up specific menus, some want to devise their own menus or add little treats to the diet to increase the child's enjoyment of meals or ability to participate in family events. Adding or changing ingredients is limited only by the mathematical confines of the ketogenic ratio and by the child's protein requirement.

Children, on or off the diet, often will ask for the same meal over and over. Because the meals are nutritionally balanced, a child can eat the same meal for breakfast, lunch, and dinner, and for many days in a row. Often, it's the parents who get tired of seeing the same thing on their child's plate and demand new meals.

Of course, fats, carbohydrates, and protein must be kept in proper balance, and enough protein must be supplied in the diet to support a child's physical development. Still, parents and dietitians can find ways to include treats for the children that are properly calculated into the diet. After all, the object of the ketogenic diet is to control seizures. Within the limits of this goal, the diet can be made as easy as possible for a child to live with.

Parents should carefully research any and all new foods they wish to introduce into the diet, especially commercially processed foods. Foods whose protein, fat, and carbohydrate content are not clearly labeled should be avoided. So-called diet foods or sugar-free foods, such as some chewing gums, may contain carbohydrates that make them inap-propriate for the diet or at least make it necessary that they be calculated in.

> **NO ADDITIONAL MEALS** should be created by parents until finetuning has been accomplished. Adding "fancy foods"just adds to the difficulty of teasing out what is wrong when ketones are low.

TIPS FOR TEENS (FROM A TEEN)

- *When using lipstick, soap, or suntan lotion, check for any kind of sugar. One time, I used some soap that had sugar in it. I didn't know that at the time though. That night I had seizures from it.*
- *When at a social event such as Youth Group, Prom, a school party, etc., focus on the socialization part of it. If the food bugs you, mingle and talk with people who are not eating food at the time.*
- *Listen to music that is inspirational to you. This should be a song that helps one know "I can do this! I'm*

not alone!" When I started the diet, my favorite song to listen to was "Hero" by Mariah Carey. It helped me sooooo much!

- Remember that even if the kids in your class or classes are eating candy, you are getting better even if it is tough. I know this issue all too well! When I was in middle and high school, the teachers would give out candy for no reason at all, and I'd be totally bummed out. However, I knew I was getting better and that thought helped me a ton!

- When asked why you don't have to eat the cafeteria food, just say something like: "I don't want to get sick!" You could even do a twist on that. Say someone says "Hey! You are soooooooooo lucky! You don't have to eat the lunch lady's food!" You could just smile and joke with them saying something like: "The Lunch lady's food is OK., but I'm getting better by not eating it."

—KM

"FREE" FOODS

No foods on the ketogenic diet are actually "free," meaning available on an unlimited basis. What are often referred to as "free" foods are those that can be eaten occasionally in small quantities without being calculated into the daily ketogenic menu plans.

Free foods include 25g of lettuce; one walnut, macadamia nut, or pecan; three filberts; or three ripe (black) olives. Most other foods, such as sugar-free Jell-O or any carbohydrate-based snack food, cannot be used at all without being calculated into the diet.

Any added foods outside of meal plans can make a difference in seizure control. Children who eat free foods every day may find that they affect seizure control. For children who continue to have seizures on the diet, free foods should be the first thing restricted during the fine-tuning process.

WHEN SHE CAME TO US, *Jennifer was tied in a wheelchair. She was so impaired by her drop seizures and her medications that* *she couldn't stand. She was already on a low-protein diet because her liver had been damaged by medication. Five days after she started the initial fast and ketogenic diet, she was running down the hall! Everybody was so excited. Back home, she didn't need naps anymore. Her anticonvulsants were stopped. She was doing well and not having any seizures. Then the seizures came back, a little bit at first and, of course, we had to recheck everything. It turned out that Jennifer liked nuts. She was allowed two "free" nuts per day. But her mother had started giving her extra nuts, seven per day, because she was begging for them, and they made her so happy. When we went back to two nuts a day the seizures came back under control.*

—MK

SPECIFIC FOODS

Initial menus for the diet are usually calculated using "generic" fruits and vegetables but designating specific meats and fats. Vegetables are placed in Group A or Group B, depending on their carbohydrate content. Group A vegetables have less carbohydrate, so the quantity of Group A vegetables in a given menu can be twice the amount of Group B vegetables. Within the generic groups, foods are interchangeable. This approach is easier for families and allows parents to pick from a list of varied fruits and vegetables.

However, the foods within these lists actually vary in content, and that variation can affect optimal seizure control for some patients. For example, 10 percent (Group B) fruits actually vary in carbohydrate content from 7g per 100g (strawberries) to over 17g per 100g (purple grapes).

Fresh meats vary even more widely. One hundredg of lean ground beef contains 24g of protein, while 100g of pork chop contains 32g of protein. One hundredg of eye round beef contains only 6.5g of fat, while 100g of lean ground beef contains about 19g of fat. For this reason, meats are not given in the form of a generic exchange list.

For many children, this level of variation is unimportant, but for some children it appears to make the difference between inadequate ketosis to control seizures and sufficient ketosis. Therefore, when a child needs fine-tuning, we try calculating the menus with exact foods instead of using generic food groups. Using the computer to calculate individual diets with specific foods can make a large difference in ketosis and therefore in seizure control.

The use of processed foods such as hot dogs and deli meats may cause a drop in urine ketones and result in a rise of seizures. The content of these foods is hard to assess. The labeling of their content is not exact. They are usually high in carbohydrates and sodium and relatively low in protein. These issues make them not only poor choices for maintaining optimum ketones but also poor for supplying adequate protein. Therefore, while fine-tuning the diet of a child with continued seizure activity, parents are requested to withhold processed foods for 1 month to see if this has an effect.

Fats

Not all fats are equal. A child who is having difficulty producing sufficient ketosis may need to have the type of fats in her diet adjusted. It may help to reduce or remove the less dense fats such as butter and mayonnaise and substitute canola, flaxseed, olive, or MCT oil (Table 8.1). Medium-chain triglyceride (MCT) oil is more efficiently metabolized, helping to produce a deeper ketosis. We use MCT oil for only a portion of the fat allowance, however, because when ingested in large quantities, it often causes gastrointestinal disturbances such as diarrhea or vomiting.

TABLE 8-1: The Protein, Carbohydrate, Fat, and Calorie Content of "Fats"(kcal)

	Grams	Protein	Fat	Carb	Kcal
Butter	100	0.67	81.33	0.00	735

Mar-garine, stick corn	100	0.00	76.00	0.00	684
Mayon-naise, Hell-man's	100	1.43	80.00	0.70	729
Corn oil	100	0.00	97.14	0.00	874
Olive oil	100	0.00	96.43	0.00	868
Canola oil	100	0.00	90.00	0.00	810
Flaxseed oil	100	0.00	100.00	0.00	900
Peanut oil	100	0.00	96.43	0.00	868
MCT oil	100	0.00	92.67	0.00	834
Safflow-er oil	100	0.00	97.14	0.00	874

We suggest using, as much as possible, unsaturated oils that contain a high fat level per gram and little or no carbohydrate or protein. Flaxseed oil is a good, heart-healthy choice. When using MCT oil, we begin with 5g per meal, or 15 totalg daily, for children who need to go into deeper ketosis. This may be increased slowly, as tolerated, until seizure control seems as good as possible with minimal side effects.

FREQUENCY OF MEALS AND SNACKS

Not only is the *quantity* of food (calories) and its *quality* (ketogenic ratio and nutritional content) important, but also the *timing* of food intake can influence the success of the ketogenic diet.

As described in Chapter 1, an individual on a normal diet stores energy for short-term use as glycogen and fat. During periods between eating or during starvation, the body first burns carbohydrate from food recently eaten, then burns carbohydrate that it has stored as glycogen, and finally begins to burn fat. Burning fat, in the absence of carbohydrate, results in ketosis.

Children on the ketogenic diet have virtually no carbohydrate in their diet, and they consume few calories, so they have virtually no stores of glycogen. Therefore, they depend on fat for their energy.

A child who is at his desirable weight has very little stored fat and therefore is dependent on the fats she eats at each meal. If too long a time passes between meals, the child may run out of fat to burn. His body will then burn some of its stored protein, but this will make his ketones decrease, and seizures may result.

__WILLIAM WAS A 3-YEAR-OLD__ who was doing very well on the diet. His seizures decreased dramatically, but his parents noticed that he continued to have a few seizures early in the morning, before he woke up. On close questioning, the dietitian discovered that the family fed William at 5:00P.M. and put him to bed at 7P.M. He didn't get up until about 7:30A.M. William's ketones always measured very low in the morning, which the ketoteam interpreted as a sign that he needed to spread out his food intake. The early morning seizures disappeared after his dietitian calculated a late-night snack into William's diet.

Children usually have breakfast in the early morning and eat lunch around noon, but dinnertime is very variable. Some children are fed supper as early as 5:30P.M. and then go to bed at 7:30 or 8:00P.M. This means that they will not have eaten for 12 to 14 hours before their breakfast. This makes little difference to a child on a normal diet, who has plenty of energy reserves stored as glycogen and fat. But a child on the ketogenic diet may not have sufficient reserves to maintain ketosis overnight. If a child eats dinner later or has a snack at bedtime, the body is less likely to run out of ketones during the night. This may help to control early-morning seizures.

NUTRASWEET

NutraSweet has been reported by some parents to induce seizures. If the parents suspect that NutraSweet is causing their child's seizures, we ask that they test this by withholding it for a week or two and observing seizure frequency when the NutraSweet is stopped. If seizure frequency increases when NutraSweet is again reintroduced, it should be avoided. Avoiding NutraSweet limits the flexibility of using readily available diet sodas, since most carbohydrate-free drinks are made with it. Parents can make drinks using saccharin instead if desired.

COMMON PROBLEMS IN THE FIRST MONTHS ON THE DIET

Weight gain

The most common error in initiating the diet is the improper estimation of a child's caloric needs. For some children, the initial estimate of calories and ratio is appropriate, or at least sufficient, and seizures are completely controlled on the diet as initially prescribed. For some children, however, overestimation of caloric needs means that, while seizures decrease after the initiation process, they are not as well controlled as they could be.

Overestimation of calories takes place partly because the recommended daily allowances (RDAs) of calories on which diet calculations are based are for average children of a given height and weight, with an average level of activity. (See Chapter 12, "Calculating the Ketogenic Diet," for more details.) However, the ketogenic diet is often used with children whose motor or intellectual capabilities are impaired to the point that they burn far fewer calories than average, healthy children.

It is tempting to start small, profoundly handicapped children on calories that are geared to more active children of the same height and weight, because a dietitian usually prefers to err on the high side than to underestimate calories. However, we often find that such children gain weight at this calorie level, and it becomes necessary to cut back. It may be preferable to take better account of the child's activity level when making the original calculations. Restricting calories for less active children results in better ketosis and earlier improvement in seizure control. It is also psychologically easier for families to add calories or a snack to the diet than to reduce calories.

An example of this was Tammy, a severely damaged 9-month-old, who was very inactive. Her only activity, in fact, was multiple flexion seizures, more than 100 per day. Her height was at only the 5th percentile, but her weight, at 24 pounds, was at the 90th percentile, possibly as the result of steroids used to treat her seizures. To get her into ketosis adequate for seizure control, she needed to be brought down closer to her desirable weight.

After a major battle with the hospital's nutrition staff over our diet prescription (they thought that our very low caloric prescription was inadequate), the ketogenic diet calculation for Tammy was set according to her basal calorie level (that needed just to maintain bodily function), 428 calories/day, about half that of an average, active 9-month-old. After 15 months on the ketogenic diet, Tammy weighed 21.5 pounds, so that her height and weight were both at the 5th percentile.

As she approached her desirable weight and had less body fat to burn to make ketones, Tammy's ketone levels began to drop and the ketogenic ratio was raised to 4:1. By the time she was 2 years old, Tammy's seizures had decreased more than 95 percent. She had seizures only rarely, during illness. It was only when Tammy's calories were very restricted that she lost weight and her seizure control improved.

---

100 calories per day=1 pound per month

If a child has lost 1 pound in 1 month, calculation reveals that approximately 100 calories should be added to the daily diet. With these additional calories, the child should gain back the lost pound in a month. Once the child's proper caloric intake is reached, the weight gain or loss stops. Remember: No two children are identical. Basal metabolic rates differ from child to child, and activity levels can differ markedly. In each case, excessive weight gain or loss indicates that caloric intake must be adjusted.

If a child is losing too much weight, the calorie level should be increased in increments of approximately 100 calories at a time (even less in small infants). When increasing calories in infants or very inactive children, it is best to increase by 25 calories every 1 to 2 weeks until you reach the desired caloric level, since too rapid an increase seems to precipitate seizures.

Enough time should pass between increments so that an evaluation can be made as to whether the child's weight has stabilized, whether seizure activity has occurred or increased, and whether hunger is under control. If it is determined that extra calories are needed, instead of recalculating all the meal plans, a snack calculated at the prescribed ratio of fat to carbohydrate and protein may be added to the diet (calculating calories and ratios is further explained in Chapter 12). Adding a ketogenic eggnog snack to the child's daily meal plan may be a convenient alternative to recalculating all the meals in the short term while adjustments to the diet are being made. Twelveg of macadamia nuts, which equals 100 calories, also make a good snack (the macadamia nuts, naturally in a 3:1

ratio, are sometimes eaten with a calculated amount of butter to achieve a 4:1 ratio).

For average people, it takes approximately 3,500 calories to gain a pound. If a child has gained 1 pound in 1 month, then 3,500 too many calories have been consumed. Dividing the calories by the number of days (31 in a typical month) reveals that the child has consumed approximately 100 extra calories each day. By recalculating the diet at about 100 fewer calories, the dietitian can stop the weight gain.

Hunger

Because the physical quantity of food on the diet (the bulk) is smaller than in a normal diet, many children feel hungry during the first week or two of the diet, until they adjust. This may be especially true of overweight children, who will have their diets calculated to include some weight loss. However, ketosis itself decreases the appetite, so children are much less likely to be hungry when consistently high levels of ketones are reached, usually within a week of starting the diet.

If a child initially complains of being hungry, try to determine whether:

- She is really hungry.
- She has not yet adapted to the smaller portion.
- She wants the pleasure and comfort of eating.

Sometimes it is not the child who is hungry at all, but rather the parents who feel pity for the child or guilt about the small portions, and who project their feelings about the diet onto the child. Other times, in the complex emotional atmosphere of diet initiation, a child's cries of hunger are actually declarations of rebellion against the parents. In any case, most children lose their feelings of hunger once they adjust to the food they are consuming and achieve consistently high ketosis.

We recommend that parents deal with hunger without trying to add extra calories to the diet, at least for the first few weeks. Tricks to modify hunger without increasing calories include:

- Drinking decaffeinated diet soda or seltzer instead of water for at least part of the liquid allotment
- Freezing drinks, such as diet orange soda mixed with cream, into popsicles
- Eating a leaf of lettuce twice a day with meals
- Eating Group A vegetables or 10 percent fruits, since greater quantities of these are allowed
- Making sure that foods, such as vegetables, are patted dry so that water is not part of the weight
- Recalculating the diet plan into four equal meals, or three meals and a snack, while maintaining a constant level of calories and the proper ketogenic ratio

THE HUNGER PARADOX Ketosis is an appetite suppressant. If reducing calories on the diet leads to better ketosis, it may decrease hunger as well. Therefore, children who are getting too many calories and gaining weight on the diet may feel hungrier than those who are getting fewer calories. Children who are hungry on

> their diet may have been given too much to eat! Therefore, *reducing calories may help to relieve hunger.*

- *Decreasing* calories slightly to raise ketosis and suppress hunger

Non-diet problems

Children who are on the diet become irritable and cry for many reasons, just as other children do. It is not always due to the diet.

Celeste, age 2, had been home from the hospital 4 days when her father called the doctor. "My wife is exhausted from staying with Celeste in the hospital," he said. "Now Celeste won't eat anything. She's crying, she's sleepy, she's whining all the time. We can't live like this!" His voice cracked with exasperation. "I can't take this diet!"

"How many seizures was she having last week, before she went into the hospital?" the doctor asked.

"More than a hundred every day."

"How many did she have during the fasting?"

"About ten a day."

"How many did she have yesterday at home?"

"One."

"Let's not give up on the diet so fast then," the doctor said. "Maybe there's a reason why she is so sleepy and irritable." On further investigation, it was discovered that Celeste had developed a fever, and her pediatrician diagnosed a urinary tract infection. Once this was treated, Celeste continued on the diet and did very well.

When problems appear in a child on the ketogenic diet, don't always assume that the diet is the cause of the problem. A child may be irritable from the hospital stay or from the difficulty of making such a radical adjustment in her life. She may rebel against the extra attention and pressure to which she is being exposed. She may be coming down with the flu or a cold. A cautious approach to fine-tuning over several weeks or months after the start of the diet will make it easier to remain on the diet.

Thirst

Thirst is not a common problem for children on the ketogenic diet, since ketones also decrease thirst. However, it is important to watch the child's urine output, particularly in hot weather, since extra fluid may be needed.

FLUID RESTRICTION is a part of the tradition of the diet, but has never been adequately studied. There may or may not be a need for fluid restriction, but at present we recommend it.

Liquid levels in the ketogenic diet are usually set at around 60cc per kilogram of body weight or approximately 1cc per calorie on the diet. One of the goals of the diet is to maintain the body in a minimally hydrated state. Liquid levels must strike a balance between being high enough for adequate body function without being so high that they adversely affect the diet. Too little liquid can result in kidney stones.

It seems important for many children to space the consumption of liquids throughout the day and not to give a thirsty child a big drink all at once, because this can sometimes cause breakthrough seizure activity and can also leave the child thirstier later on. Some parents give their child a regular dose of water or diet soda (with no caffeine) every 1 to 2 hours during the day. Other children seem to be able to drink larger amounts of liquid with no seizures.

In hot climates or during summer months, the cream in the diet need not be counted as part of the allotted liquid. In effect, this raises the liquid allowance by the quantity of the cream.

A child may become dehydrated if the fluid allowance is insufficient. Signs of dehydration include dry lips and skin, infrequent urination, sunken eyes, and lethargy. Most thirst problems, as well as problems of excessive acidosis, can be corrected by increasing fluid intake, usually in increments of 10 to 20cc/kg of body weight per day until the problem is corrected. The ketoteam can determine adequate fluid replacement levels and ongoing fluid requirements by monitoring a child's weight, urine quantity, specific gravity of the urine, and ketone levels.

Kidney stones

Painful kidney stones occur in as many as one in six children on the ketogenic diet, probably partially as a result of inadequate fluid intake. To help children avoid developing kidney stones, we ask parents to test the child's urine once a week with a Hematest dipstick for specific gravity and blood. (Hematest assesses blood and other substances in the urine. Since they are more expensive than the Ketostix, we suggest using them only once a week.) If blood is detected in the urine, a child is instructed to drink freely for 48 hours, following which the fluid allotment is increased. If blood in the urine persists despite this increase in fluid, a urine sample is sent to a lab, where tests for calcium, creatinine, and uric acid levels, as well as reagent strip analysis and microanalysis are conducted.

A renal sonogram may be necessary if the calcium to creatinine ratio is above 0.2mg and/or the urine remains positive for blood. If a kidney stone is found, the child is started on Bicitra or Polycitra K to alkalinize the urine and dissolve the crystals. With alkalinization, even established stones may disappear. This has never been proven, but we have found it to be a helpful therapy. If stones do not resolve with this treatment, lithotripsy or, on rare occasions, even surgical removal of kidney stones may be necessary.

Other signs of possible kidney stones include sharp abdominal pain and nonspecific illness with fever, poor appetite, or an unexplained increase in seizures. In a child on the ketogenic diet, an otherwise unexplained increase in seizures may be due to kidney stones.

Sleepiness and sedation

On the ketogenic diet, excess sleepiness or lethargy can be due to excessive ketosis or medication toxicity. Medication levels frequently rise in the blood of children on the ketogenic diet even without a change in dosage. The rise may be due to the partial dehydration state, to altered serum binding of the drug to the blood proteins, to elevated drug levels in the brain, or to changes in drug metabolism. Medication levels should be monitored carefully during the fasting and diet-initiation period, and those medications that are likely to cause drowsiness, such as phenobarbital and benzodiazepines, should be decreased if sleepiness occurs.

Some children on the diet who have lab results showing medications at therapeutic levels but who exhibit signs of medication toxicity may improve when the drug dose is lowered. Drugs are bound to blood proteins and, when the child is acidotic, as they are on the diet, less of the drug is bound up, and more of the drug gets into the brain to cause sleepiness. Although fasting and diet initiation can cause lethargy, the symptoms should rarely persist beyond 2 to 3 weeks.

Some children become more alert and energetic while on the ketogenic diet. This may be a result of taking fewer medications or having fewer seizures. As mentioned in Chapter 9, hypoglycemia or low blood sugar levels can also cause lethargy during the initial fasting period, but blood sugar levels should return to near normal within a few days of starting the diet.

Constipation

Constipation can become a problem because of the small volume of food, low fiber content, reduced fluid intake, and high concentration of fat in this diet. Constipation may cause stomach pains and discomfort. Fortunately, it does not have to be an obstacle to continuing the diet. Using Group A vegetables in meal plans can help increase the bulk and fiber in the diet a little bit. Also, two leaves of lettuce, or about one-half cup of chopped lettuce, are allowed each day as so-called "free" food.

Make sure that the child is receiving the proper amount of liquid. Increasing daily liquid levels by 100 to 150cc may help combat constipation.

If a child continues to have problems with constipation, laxatives, stool softeners, or enemas may help. MiraLax™ powder is often effective.

Full-strength enemas should not be used regularly because they can affect the lining of the intestine. Small amounts of Colace (1% solution or suppository), Milk of Magnesia, Epsom salts, or MCT oil calculated into the diet might be effective in maintaining bowel regularity and preventing constipation. Fleets enemas and aloe vera are also useful. All laxatives must be sugar-free.

CHANGING THE DIET'S KETOGENIC RATIO

Raising the diet's ratio (fat-to-(protein+carbohydrate)) increases the amount of fats consumed, with the goal of increasing ketosis and thereby resulting in better seizure control. If a child is continuing to have seizures, and if careful, thorough sleuthing has not revealed a cause, then raising the ketogenic ratio may be considered. We raise ratios in half-point increments, from 3:1 to 3.5:1, or from 4:1 to 4.5:1.

A 5:1 ketogenic ratio can occasionally be used for a few months, but it is so restrictive and so barely nutritionally adequate that we do not maintain it for more than a 6-month period. We prefer the lowest ratio adequate to produce deep ketosis and seizure control.

Occasionally, the ratio is decreased during the fine-tuning period if a child becomes anorexic and will not eat; if she remains too acidotic; if she is experiencing frequent illnesses; or if she is having digestive difficulties on the diet. Most older children start the diet on a 4:1 ratio. They are then adjusted down slowly after their first year on the diet.

Overweight children are an exception to this rule. We frequently start them on a diet in 3:1 ratio with restricted calories to facilitate weight loss. As they lose weight, they burn their own body fat, and this produces high ketones for them. As they approach their desirable weight, overweight children have less of their own body fat to burn, so we may need to increase the ratio to maintain the same high level of ketones. Adolescents often need a 3:1 ratio to provide sufficient protein within their caloric restrictions. Very young children are also usually started on a 3:1 diet to allow more protein for their growth.

MEDICATION LEVELS

The fine-tuning period usually involves adjusting medication levels as well as food and other nonfood factors. Unless a child displays signs of overmedication, it is preferable to wait several weeks after initiation before beginning to taper any medications. Only one medication should be tapered at a time, and diet changes should not be made at the same time as medication changes.

Phenobarbital is the one known exception. Phenobarbital is bound to protein in the blood and, when the body becomes acidotic, more is unbound and gets into the brain. Therefore, we usually decrease the dose of the child's phenobarbital by one-third when the fasting is commenced.

It is not uncommon for one or even a few breakthrough seizures to occur 24 to 72 hours after each decrease in medication dose. Parents and physicians should not reintroduce the medication or take any other action unless the seizures continue for more than a week. If the increase in seizures continues for a week, reintroduction of the medication may be necessary. Benzodiazepines such as clonazepam are addictive, and their withdrawal commonly produces seizures. For this reason, their reduction must be done very gradually to minimize withdrawal symptoms. A compounding pharmacy may be useful in preparing the increasingly dilute, sugar-free solutions needed for the weaning process.

Reducing anticonvulsant medications is a secondary but important goal of the ketogenic diet. Some children on the diet are able to stop taking all anticonvulsant medications and never have to go on them again. The situation varies for each individual.

Don't be in too much of a hurry to decrease or eliminate medications. Get the diet working first. Get the seizures under better control first. When the family and child are on a stable routine, one medicine at a time can be gradually reduced and, if no recurrence of seizures occurs, eliminated. If medication is reduced in this systematic, gradual fashion and the child does have a few seizures, it becomes easy to figure out the reason. The key to weaning children off their anticonvulsant medications during the fine-tuning period is to separate the effects of decreasing doses of medications from other factors in the diet. In other words, don't reduce medications at the same time as adjusting the food. Also, if a child has breakthrough seizures while the medicine is being reduced, don't assume that the seizures are a result of the tapering off. Look for all the possible factors and try to determine whether the reduction in medication is the cause.

THE LIMITS OF FINE-TUNING

Not every child becomes seizure-free on the ketogenic diet. Not every child becomes medication-free. After working carefully with the ketoteam for several months, you will have to decide if there is enough improvement in your child's seizures, in his drug toxicity, in his life and in your life to continue trying to make the diet even better. If you decide, together with the dietitian, that the child has received as much benefit from the diet as possible, then you will have to decide if that is good enough to continue. You can always go back to medication. Returning to the medication will virtually always result in re-control of the seizures.

The decision tree

The first thing to look for when breakthrough seizures occur is whether the child has had an opportunity to eat something not on the diet. Someone may have given food or the child may have helped himself. One child was found to be sneaking sugared toothpaste in an upstairs bathroom. Another was slipping out of bed at night and raiding the refrigerator. Another girl had a seizure on Sunday, and her mother found to her dismay that a well-meaning grown-up at church had given her a lollipop.

Another possible cause of breakthrough activity on the diet is a calorie level that is set too high. If the body takes in more calories than are needed for maintenance, it will store those extra calories as fat. The body must burn all calories taken in to produce adequate ketosis and seizure control. Remember, the diet is simulating starvation, and you can't store calories when starving. As few as 100 calories too many per day can upset ketosis. In smaller infants, even 25 calories per day may be critical.

The level of urinary ketosis may vary with the time of day. It is usually lower in the morning and higher later in the day. This natural variation in the level of ketones as measured in the urine does not necessarily indicate a problem if it is not accompanied by seizures.

At times, we test the system in a child with low ketones by fasting the child for 24 hours. If the ketones rise after this fast, then we decrease calories. With the exception of weight gain correlated to growth in height, weight gain on the diet is an indication that calorie levels are set too high. At an excess of 100 calories per day, it takes an entire month before any weight gain is seen. Therefore, some caloric adjustments can be made based on low ketone levels.

Sometimes better control may be achieved by using a 4.5:1 ratio or even a 5:1 ratio for a period of time. The higher the diet ratio, the more restricted food options get, so the implications of raising the diet ratio should be seriously considered before it is prescribed.

EXCESS KETOACIDOSIS occurs with 15 percent to 20 percent of our children starting the diet and may require either IV fluids or fluids given by a nasogastric tube for the first several days.

The most common cause of breakthrough seizures in a child who is getting the proper food and liquid levels is illness or fever.

An isolated seizure during illness requires no action on the part of the parents. Repeated breakthrough seizures can be the presenting sign of kidney stones, urinary tract infection, gastroenteritis, or other childhood infections. See Chapter 11 for greater detail on managing acute illness during the diet.

The ketogenic diet decision tree in Figure 8.1 can be used as a guide to investigating breakthrough seizures.

A 100 PERCENT SOLUTION MAY NOT EXIST

Improvements in behavior, mood, mental alertness, and a general sense of well-being are additional benefits that the diet often brings. If parents set a goal of total seizure control, they may be setting themselves up for disappointment. Total control may not be possible.

After trying the diet for the initial 3-month period, and after working with the ketoteam to figure out if greater control can be achieved by adjusting food or medications, parents of children who have not responded to the diet or who have improved only moderately must make a decision. These parents must weigh the benefits of the diet for their child against its burdens. Then they have to decide whether it is worthwhile for them to continue on the diet.

FIGURE 8-1

The Ketogenic Diet Decision Tree—for when a child with previous control begins having seizures

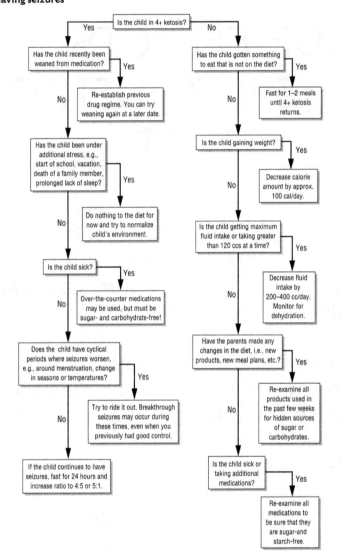

CHAPTER NINE

SIDE EFFECTS OF THE KETOGENIC DIET

All therapies (and even some everyday products) have either side effects or potential side effects. For example: Too much water can cause convulsions, and aspirin may cause ulcers. The side effects of most medical treatments are of two sorts: allergic or dose-related. Anticonvulsant medications can cause both allergic and dose-related side effects.

The allergic side effects of anticonvulsant medication may include rashes, which can progress to a condition termed Stevens-Johnson syndrome that produces sores in the mouth, rashes on the skin, involvement of the liver and kidneys, and even death. While uncommon, the Stevens-Johnson syndrome can occur with any anticonvulsant medication, and every individual taking anticonvulsants should be alert to the possibility of this condition. Isolated problems with individual organ systems may also occur.

The toxic (or dose-related) side effects of anticonvulsant medications are usually related to the dose of the drug or the way it is metabolized. These potential side effects include fatigue, sedation, cognitive impairment, and problems with coordination. A parent should be aware of changes in a child's function and make the physician aware of them. Because virtually all problems are related to the dose of a drug or its metabolism, these problems are usually corrected by lowering the dose or eliminating that drug. Interactions between medications may also result in the toxicity of one or the other.

The ketogenic diet also has side effects and complications, but far fewer than those of anticonvulsant medications. Because the diet consists of normal foods, no allergic side effects occur. All the side effects or complications of the ketogenic diet are related to the metabolic changes that it induces. Although there may potentially be very long-term problems due to having been on the diet, none have been documented.

PROBLEMS DURING THE START OF THE KETOGENIC DIET

Although many minor problems may arise during the induction of the diet, we do not find any of them to be serious side effects, and all are easily managed.

Sleepiness

Fasting for 36 hours may lead to hypoglycemia. For this reason, children are fasted in the hospital where they can be observed. Blood sugars of 30 to 40 are not uncommon and virtually never require a medical response. If blood sugars of less than 30 are found, the test is repeated in 1 hour. If a child is symptomatic—too sleepy or sweaty—30cc of orange juice may be given and repeated in 30 minutes if necessary.

We avoid testing that requires sedation during this time to avoid possible confusion with hypoglycemia. The acidosis that occurs during fasting may change the binding of certain anticonvulsants, most notably phenobarbital top serum protein, therefore allowing higher concentration into the brain. This results in lethargy in some children. The sedation of the fasting helps many of the children and their families to get through these 36 hours.

Dehydration

The ketosis associated with fasting decreases thirst as well as causing sedation, therefore fluid intake may be suboptimal. We encourage families to get the allotted fluids into their child, but if the child shows signs of dehydration, an IV or a bolus of carbohydrate-free fluids given by nasogastric (NG) tube may be useful.

Vomiting

Excess ketosis and acidosis (a bicarbonate level of less than 10 mEq/L or a pH <7.2) may result in vomiting. If the vomiting is repeated and is accompanied by sedation, an IV with carbohydrate-free fluids, sometimes with a small bolus of added sugar will stop the vomiting.

Refusal to eat at the end of the fast

The diet is first introduced as an eggnog with one-third of the future daily allotment of calories. This is subsequently increased to two-thirds, then to the full diet. Most children scarf it down in a blink. Some are too ketotic and lack hunger. These need encouragement. The eggnog can be taken as a shake, may be frozen as ice cream, or microwaved to make "scrambled eggs." Because each sip is equal in content, the eggnog may be sipped over several hours.

PROBLEMS DURING THE DIET

Weight gain or weight loss

The most common side effect of the diet is weight gain or loss. This is not a serious side effect, but to assure optimal seizure control and ketosis, optimal weight should be achieved and maintained. Checking weight weekly can assess changes and allow correction of the proper caloric management. Weight gain and loss are further discussed in Chapter 8.

Infections and illness

All children suffer intermittent illnesses, even those on the ketogenic diet. No good evidence suggests that children on the diet are more susceptible to infections than others. As discussed in Chapter 8, during illness, a child may become dehydrated and require fluids or become too ketotic or too acidotic. These conditions are usually manifested as vomiting, sleepiness, or rapid deep breathing. If a child reaches such a state, an ounce of orange juice (which may be repeated), can usually break the excess ketosis. If it continues, IV fluids may be required. These manifestations of illness are not reasons to discontinue the diet.

Growth

Children grow normally in height on the ketogenic diet, although younger children appear to grow at a somewhat slower rate than usual. It is speculated, but unproven, that when the diet is discontinued, growth catches up. Growth in weight is, as has been previously discussed, carefully monitored to maintained ideal body mass. When growth is a problem, we often lower the ratio to allow more protein.

Vitamin deficiency

The ketogenic diet is deficient in vitamins and perhaps in minerals as well. We have produced a case of beri beri due to lack of thiamin and seen reports of cases of optic neuritis due to the same deficiency. Selenium deficiency also has been reported. All children on the ketogenic diet should receive multivitamin and mineral supplements.

Kidney stones

Kidney stones are not uncommon and may be initially manifested as an increase in seizures, nonspecific illness, fever, poor appetite, and occasionally an increase in abdominal pain. Unlike adults, in children these stones do not often seem to cause pain, but may, if unrecognized, grow sufficiently large to require lithotripsy or even surgical removal. It is best to recognize the propensity to stones or their early formation.

Kidney stones are usually either calcium stones or uric-acid stones. For the early detection of stones, parents are asked to check the urine weekly for traces of blood with Hematest, as discussed in Chapter 8. We also check the child's urine episodically for its calcium/creatine ratio. If this ratio is above 0.2 and/or the urine remains positive for blood, then Bicitra or Polycitra is added to the diet to alkalinize the urine and solubilize the stones. The fluid allotment is also increased. These latter measures are often sufficient to dissolve the stones. Rarely, lithotripsy or even surgical removal of the stones is necessary. Kidney stones are rarely such a problem, or so difficult to manage, that a successful diet needs to be discontinued.

Pancreatitis has been reported and, while uncommon, can be serious. The symptoms are similar to those of kidney stones and may be related to elevated cholesterol and lipids. A decrease in the diet ratio may be useful in allowing a child with pancreatitis to remain on the diet.

Hypercholesteremia, lipid abnormalities, and atherosclerosis

Abnormalities of lipid metabolism are the concerns of cardiologists and lipid specialists when they hear that a child is eating a diet of 80 percent fat. They have preached the dangers of eating fat for so long that they believe children who eat a lot of fat will all develop atherosclerosis and have strokes and heart attacks. However, when a high-fat diet, such as the ketogenic diet, is accompanied by caloric restriction, no weight gain occurs and the changes in the lipids, cholesterol, LDL, and lipoproteins are slight.

Our study of the lipid changes in children on the ketogenic diet indicates that, while some elevation of cholesterol and changes in lipoproteins occurs to "levels that exceed current recommendations for normal children," the significance of these levels is unclear. The change is usually about one-third higher than the child's starting cholesterol. Often, the diet is discontinued in 2 years or less, and the child returns to a normal lower-fat diet. Presumably, the lipids return to normal. In a study of children on the diet for over 6 years, most of them had cholesterol in the normal range (average 201mg/dL), suggesting this is true.

Very high levels of lipid abnormalities have occasionally been found, with cholesterol levels of

1,000mg and serum hyperlipidemia. In several of these patients, we found familial hyperlipidemia, which was exacerbated by the high-fat diet. Reduction of the diet ratio has allowed these children to remain on the diet and maintain normal lipid levels. Occasionally, we also increase the percentage of polyunsaturated fats to lower the lipids as well. At our center, it is virtually never necessary for a child to discontinue the diet due to lipid changes.

Although theoretical concerns exist, no studies have been made of the long-term effects of the ketogenic diet on strokes or cardiac problems, and no evidence suggests long-term effects of these lipid abnormalities.

Death

Deaths have been reported by various authors, several due to a cardiomyopathy, one questionably due to selenium deficiency. Others were secondary to lipoid pneumonia. In more than 500 children, we have seen one death, due to the recurrence of a cardiomyopathy of unknown nature, which started well before the diet. We also have seen two children who died one day *before* starting the diet, emphasizing the very fragile and desperate nature of some of these children. We are unaware of other deaths of children on the ketogenic diet, and are uncertain of the relationship, if any, of death to the diet.

OTHER ALLEGED COMPLICATIONS

Bleeding disorders, bruising, basal ganglia changes, changes in gamma globulin, an increase in infections, lipoid pneumonia due to aspiration of the liquid diet, and doubtless other problems have been reported as occurring in children on the diet. What, if any, relationship the diet has to these problems remains unclear, and most of these reports discuss only one or two children. Some evidence suggests decreased bone density, and children on the diet for over 6 years appear to be at higher risk for bone fractures. This risk must be carefully watched in any child on the ketogenic diet, but this loss of bone mass also occurs with many anticonvulsant drugs.

However, it is notable that even those who catalogue these events find the diet safe and effective. One must keep these complications in mind and weigh these potential risks against the risks of continuing seizures and of the continued use of new anticonvulsants.

CHAPTER TEN

MAKING IT WORK AT HOME AND ON THE ROAD

> **BE CREATIVE,** but follow the rules exactly.
>
> Follow the rules exactly, but be creative.

As long as you follow the rules exactly, but think creatively, you and your child can do just about anything you ever did before the diet started.

TIME SAVERS

At first, most families find that the diet is very time-consuming to plan and prepare. But it gets faster and easier as you become accustomed to using the gram scale and planning meals in advance. We have estimated that, in the first weeks, shopping and meal preparation may add an extra hour or two of commitment each day. But after this initial period, once you have gotten used to weighing food, parents say that preparing the diet may add a half-hour per day at most.

THE FIRST TIME, SHOPPING TAKES FOREVER. Going up and down the aisles reading the fine print on each label, searching for the words ending in "ose" or "ol" almost made me give up! But the second time was easier. Then I learned the brands I could use, and I only had to check to see that they hadn't changed the ingredients.
—KM

Preparing and storing meals or parts of meals in advance can save much time. You can refrigerate many foods for a few days or freeze them for a week or more. The following are some time-saving tips from parents who have experienced the diet:

- I cut up his favorite vegetables and keep them in plastic bags in the refrigerator for a few days. Then I can take them out and weigh a meal in no time.

- I usually make cream popsicles once a week. He has one after every dinner.
- We measure a day or two of meals at a time and put them in containers. That way we only have to do the weighing about every other day. Also, we can either serve the meals at home or take them with us if we are eating out.
- Whenever someone is celebrating a birthday at school, I know what to make for him—I send him in with a fruittopped ketogenic cheesecake so he can have something good to eat, too.
- I put a cream shake in a container and freeze it, so that he can eat it later as ice cream or let it thaw back down to a shake.
- I always keep some tuna or chicken salad and bags of cut-up vegetables stored in the refrigerator in case I can't be there to fix dinner myself. He also takes these stored meals to school.
- Be certain to label each meal or each part of a meal (Monday bkfst, Wed. sup) before putting it in the

refrigerator or the freezer, so that you remember what goes together.

GOING TO SCHOOL AND OTHER SHORT TRIPS

Anything the family did before, they can still do on the diet—it will just take a little more planning. Every parent who has been through the diet has suggestions to offer:

- The key to making the diet "portable" is reusable storage containers.
- Cold food is easier to transport than hot food.
- It is easy to get food microwaved in a restaurant.
- It is usually easier to weigh and assemble a whole meal or several meals at home in advance than to weigh food on the road.

WITH BOTH OF US WORKING, and with all of the sports and church things for the other kids, finding time to make Brian's ketogenic meals was very hard. We finally found that if his mom and I worked together on

Saturday morning, we could make all the meals for the week, label them, and put them in the freezer. Then, at night, we only had to make the family's supper—his was all ready to microwave.

—KD

Eggnog is the traditional replacement meal, designed for all-purpose substitution in case of travel, sickness, or emergencies that make it difficult to prepare a meal. Eggnog is a complete meal-in-one (except for vitamin supplements), which is part of what makes it so convenient. Most children like the taste. Each sip is ketogenically balanced, so they don't have to drink all of it, or drink it all at once, to get its ketogenic effect.

Macadamia nuts, sometimes mixed with butter to achieve a higher ratio (they are naturally 3:1), can also be used as a meal-in-a-pinch or a travel meal or snack. A bag of chopped macadamia nuts eaten with a diet soda can be a very socially acceptable way for older children to eat around their friends, for example on a field trip or sleepover.

Neither eggnog nor macadamia nuts has enough protein or the nutritional value of regular meals containing meats, fruits, and vegetables. These are meant for snacks and should be used infrequently in place of meals. Both eggnog and macadamia nuts, however, can be extremely useful in a pinch.

WE CARRIED A SMALL COOLER WITH AN ICE PACK in it everywhere. In the morning, we fixed the whole day's meals before going out. It got so that, even if we weren't going anywhere, we would set up all the meals for the day and stick them in Tupperware containers in the refrigerator. If we were going on a long trip, we would take about 2 days' worth of food with us in the cooler and bring our scale. Also, we always carried extra ingredients that we knew might be hard to buy, like olives. Everyone has a microwave, even on airplanes. We could give a fancy restaurant a couple of Tupperware containers and instructions for how long to cook things, and they would bring the food out on their own plate. Everybody was really cooperative.

—RZ

The following are some meal ideas for taking to school or on short outings. Each meal requires several reusable containers for storage.

- Tuna, chicken, or egg salad with mayonnaise

  Fresh vegetables (cucumber, carrot, cherry tomato, celery) Sugar-free Jell-O with whipped cream
- Celery or cucumber boats stuffed with tuna salad, cream cheese and butter, or peanut butter and butter Vanilla cream shake, whipped and frozen overnight
- Sandwich rolled in lettuce (chicken, cheese, turkey, or roast beef with mayonnaise)

  Water-packed canned peaches

  Chocolate milk (cream diluted with water and flavored with pure chocolate extract and saccharin)
- Cottage cheese with chopped fruit or vegetables and mayonnaise

Cream shake, whipped and frozen overnight

- Fruit-topped "cheesecake," frozen overnight: a one-dish meal

Foods frozen overnight and taken out in the morning soften to a pudding-like consistency by lunchtime. Foods to be taken to school or on short outings can be wrapped in foil or carried in a thermal pouch or cooler for extra insulation to help stay either warm or cold. Whipped cream can be stored for a few hours and still keep its body.

__WHEN WE WENT TO DISNEYLAND,__ we just took a big cooler with three whole days of meals in labeled containers. Once we let him get a hot dog from the stand (which we then weighed), so he could feel like he was having a special treat. I wouldn't say it was easy doing all that planning, but for us it wasn't too difficult.

—RZ

If you are going out to eat at a restaurant, and you want your child to have a hot meal, call first to make sure the restaurant has a microwave that can be used for heating your food. If you are giving the child a cold meal, ask the restaurant to bring out an extra plate, which will make the food look nice and add to the feeling of family togetherness. McDonald's will usually give a cup into which you can pour a sugar-free nocalorie soda. Bring your own can or bottle of soda, because diet drinks from the fountain may contain sorbitol.

DIET DON'TS

One mother kept her child out of school for a year and hired an in-home teacher because she did not want him to be tempted by seeing other children eat. Another family stopped going out entirely—no more McDonald's, no more Sunday dinners at grandma's—until the child himself finally begged them, explaining that he would enjoy the atmosphere and would not be too tempted by the food. Another mother fed her child earlier and in another room, so he "wouldn't feel different" from his siblings. We believe it is better to aim for inclusiveness, for living as normally as possible given the diet's restrictions. In our experience, most children are able to participate in the game of making the diet as much as possible part of a normal, enjoyable life.

MANAGING ACUTE ILLNESS DURING THE DIET

It may be difficult for a child who is sick to maintain ketosis. Sick children often do not feel like eating. Their activity level changes, and they don't burn as many calories when they are ill. For these and other reasons, many children on the diet experience a decrease in their urine ketone levels when sick. Seizure activity may increase at these times, or breakthrough seizures may occur even in children who have been well controlled on the diet. Parents can rest assured that ketosis will become reestablished as the illness resolves. But seizures during illness are not solely due to a decrease in ketosis. For reasons that are not understood, children who have seizures and have never been on the diet are more likely to have a seizure during their illness.

HELPING YOUR CHILD to recover from an acute illness is more important than maintaining ketosis during times of illness!

It may be necessary to break ketosis in order to treat an illness effectively. The most important thing is to get your child well again. The ketosis can be resumed once your child is well. The following are general guidelines for caring for a sick child on the ketogenic diet.

Vomiting or diarrhea

- Give only sugar-free clear liquids. Do not worry about restricting fluids. Offer fluids as frequently as tolerated.
- If vomiting lasts for more than 24 hours, use unflavored Pedialyte™ to maintain electrolytes. Use for up to 24 hours (but not longer).
- When vomiting stops, you can introduce a one-third quantity eggnog meal. Each sip has the proper ketogenic ratio, and it is not necessary for your child to finish

the eggnog if she does not want to. Increase as tolerated until the child is eating the full diet quantity. Then resume regular menus.

- If your child becomes dehydrated and IV fluids are required, make sure that they are sugar-free (normal saline, no dextrose). Physicians and nurses in emergency rooms are not thinking about the effects that glucose in the IV might have on the diet and on the child's seizures. If blood glucose is below 40, a single bolus of glucose (1g per kilogram of body weight) may be given.

- If your child is using MCT oil in her diet, discontinue it until the illness is resolved. Substitute 1g canola or corn oil for eachg of MCT oil. The MCT oil can be resumed when your child is well.

Fever

- Give sugar-free fever-reducing medicine. Acetaminophen suppositories are an excellent fever reducer that won't interfere with the diet.

- Offer sugar-free liquids without restriction while your child has a fever.
- If an antibiotic is needed, make sure it is sugar-and sorbitolfree. Speak with your pediatrician about using injectable antibiotics when possible, because a 7-to 10-day course of oral antibiotics may interfere with ketosis.

Too much ketosis

Sometimes a change in the diet or illness can cause children to get into too much ketosis. Some signs of too much ketosis are:

- Rapid, panting (Kussmaul) breathing
- Irritability
- Increased heart rate
- Facial flushing
- Unusual fatigue or lethargy
- Vomiting

If you suspect your child may be in too much ketosis, give him 2 tablespoons of orange juice. If the symptoms persist 20 minutes after giving the juice, give a second dose of 2 tablespoons orange juice. If the second dose of juice does not improve your child's condition, call your pediatrician and the supervising physician of your child's ketogenic diet immediately.

If you cannot reach the doctors, take your child to the emergency room. The emergency room doctors will check how acidotic your child has become. Intravenous fluids or even a dose of IV glucose may be needed to break up the excessive ketosis. In the meantime, ask the emergency room to continue trying to contact your ketoteam.

Sugar-free medication

Work with your pediatrician and local pharmacist to obtain any necessary medications in sugar-free and carbohydrate-free form. A list of medications is provided in Appendix A. If a medication you need is not commercially available in carbohydrate-free form, try contacting a compounding pharmacy in your area for custom-made medications.

BABY-SITTERS AND OTHER PARENTLESS MEALS

In most households, the person who usually prepares the meals is occasionally unavailable—working late, sick, at a party, or otherwise engaged. Not to worry! With a little planning, someone else can easily put a meal together from your prepared ingredients.

Many parents store measured ingredients or prepared food a couple of days ahead of time in the refrigerator, even when they are planning to be present to prepare each meal. The habit of preparing meals in advance both saves time on a routine basis and makes it easier to cope with special situations. Just as with nonketogenic meals, it rarely hurts to have something ready in the freezer.

Some items can be measured and stored or frozen up to a week in advance:

- Popsicles
- Beef
- Sugar-free Jell-O
- Cream shakes

- Chicken
- Cut-up fresh vegetables
- Cheesecake
- Eggnog
- Ice cream

Note that foods such as ice cream must be calculated and carefully labeled to go with a particular meal that you plan to make. This is because different meal plans use varying amounts of cream, and ingredients such as fruit or oil may need to be frozen into the ice cream, depending on what else is being served for supper.

Other foods can be prepared, weighed, and stored in the refrigerator 1 or 2 days in advance:

- Cooked meat or chicken portions
- D-Zerta gelatin
- Tuna, egg, or chicken salads
- Vegetables
- Cream portions for whipping
- Fresh fruit
- Tomato sauce
- Sliced or grated cheese

If a parent sets out measured ingredients and instructions, a sibling or baby-sitter can easily carry out final assembly of the meal. Make these meals simple: Try to think of meals that can be put in one microwave dish and cooked or reheated (stew, squash/cheese/butter casserole) or meals that do not need cooking at all (tuna salad).

LONG TRIPS

Yes, the family can take vacations. Longer trips, by necessity, involve more planning than shorter ones. Many families who take long vacations choose to stay in places where they can cook, such as friends' condominiums or motels with kitchenettes, rather than in hotels. They sometimes take eggnog for the road instead of a solid meal. They take their scale, and call ahead to make sure that places where they will be staying have heavy cream and a microwave available. With the scale, they can order grilled chicken, steamed vegetables, and mayonnaise and create a quick meal right at the restaurant.

Families take coolers full of prepared ingredients for the first couple days of a trip, and perhaps staples such as artificial sweetener and mayonnaise. If they are staying in a hotel with no kitchen, they might take a camping stove to cook on. They take a lot of storage containers.

They take their calcium and multivitamin supplements, too, of course, because they never forget those.

Apart from the nuisance of planning, the diet should be no obstacle to family fun. There is no reason why a child should not live a rich, full, and healthy life while on the ketogenic diet. There is no reason to deprive yourself or the rest of the family either.

HE SKIED THIS YEAR for the first time in ages. He skied like you wouldn't believe. He's swimming, he's playing ball. He's definitely had a happier life on the diet.

—CC

BE CREATIVE

Being creative can mean compensating for a small quantity of cucumbers and carrots by slicing them in tall, thin strips and fanning them out to cover more plate space. It can mean dressing up the cream as a toasted almond ice cream, whipped into a mound, flavored with almond extract and sweetener, and sprinkled with a crushed almond. Let the child sprinkle on the nuts for fun.

There are lots of calorie-free ways to keep the food lively. Play with variables that add interest, not calories:

- Shapes
- Natural food colors or food coloring
- Herbs and spices (just a tiny pinch because these have carbohydrates)
- Pure flavoring extracts
- Pretending

Of course, many children do not care about variety and whimsy in their food. Some children are comforted by regularity. We have seen many families cook the same six meals over and over for 2 years, and the child was perfectly content.

WE FREEZE HIS DIET DECAFFEINATED POP in miniature ice cube trays. They make refreshing little treats. He has a small amount as a goodie before bedtime. We give it to him in a wine glass to make it fancy and special. We also make popsicles out of his pop. If it's clear pop, we let him mix in food coloring drops, so he is not only involved but also learning. This adds lots of laughs when his teeth and lips turn green or blue or purple.

—EH

Peaches can be swapped for strawberries, broccoli for spinach. Combine fruits or vegetables for variety—peaches with a couple of raspberries on top, or asparagus with carrots. Switching the foods around helps add variety to the meals. If a child wants variety, there's plenty of room for creativity within the diet.

HE HAS HIS SPECIAL "PIZZA." *It's just cheese and ground beef melted on a thin slice of tomato, cut into triangles the shape of pizza slices. But he loves it. It's pizza to him!*

—EH

FOLLOW THE RULES EXACTLY

If the rules are followed exactly, the family knows that the child was given the best possible chance to obtain the maximum benefits of the diet. Being very strict helps the ketoteam know where a child stands with the diet. The effect of the ketogenic diet is directly related to the food that is eaten and the liquid that is drunk. This may seem obvious, but it is the factor that makes the diet work.

Especially when using commercial products, knowing the precise content of the food is essential. Buy the exact brand specified by the dietitian. The same product, such as bologna, made by different manufacturers, may have very different proportions of protein, fat, and carbohydrates. The dietitian will have based diet calculations on the proportions of a given brand, so if a new brand is used, the calculations may have to be changed.

ABOUT A WEEK AFTER HE STARTED THE DIET, *my son was*

doing great. Then we went to the store and bought some commercial turkey loaf. The meal plan called for turkey, so we thought turkey loaf would be just as good. Well, I don't know what was in it, but my son had a very bad day the next day. That's when we discovered that, when the meal plan says turkey, it means plain, fresh turkey, not turkey loaf. You have to follow instructions to the letter.

—FD

If a different brand must be introduced, the parents or dietitian must research the product carefully, even if it means calling the manufacturer to find out. Make sure that the new brand is properly calculated into the meal plans.

IT WOULD NEVER HAVE OCCURRED *to us to eat something that wasn't allowed on the diet. Even when we were allowed to, when the diet was ending, we had a hard time imagining eating food that hadn't been allowed before.*

—CC

Even when a commercial product is known and used regularly, formulations and commercial recipes can change. If breakthrough seizures develop, this should be one source of suspicion. At the risk of repeating ourselves, the ingredients of commercially prepared foods, which are beyond your power to control, must be watched very carefully. Be cautious in reading labels as well. By law, products that contain less than 1g of an ingredient per serving may be listed as zero, so a product that you thought had no carbohydrates may actually have up to 0.9g. If used on a regular basis, this can add up to a lot of excess carbohydrates.

With basic ingredients such as fresh meat, fruit, and vegetables, this is not much of a problem, although the exact content of even fresh produce does vary slightly from one source to another.

If your child is having problems with the diet, always consider the food—both its quantity and its content—as the most likely culprit:

• Are there commercial products in the diet?

- Has the source of cream or bacon changed?
- Is the cream still 36 percent to 40 percent fat?

Different children have different amounts of tolerance for variations in food content. The little things often spell the difference between success and failure of the diet. If your child is doing well on the diet, obviously you shouldn't worry. You should simply continue to be careful.

THERE WAS ONE TIME WE WANTED TO TRY *a new brand of sausage. We read the label very carefully and checked it with Mrs. Kelly and everything. But shortly after we started including it in her diet, our daughter began feeling shaky, what she described as "wobbly" inside. Dr. Freeman said it sounded like she might be trying to break through with seizures. We're pretty sure it was because of that sausage; either the label was wrong or it referred to raw quantities and we were using cooked, or something. We went* *back to the old brand, and then she was fine.*

—MH

GET THE WHOLE FAMILY INVOLVED

When you and your child are making the tremendous effort to stick to the diet in pursuit of a tremendous goal, you need everyone's cooperation and encouragement. You can weigh the food in advance, but if you are not there at dinnertime, someone else—an older sister or brother, a sitter, a grandmother—can put it in the microwave and serve the meal.

A child on the diet and all the child's sisters and brothers, relatives, friends, and teachers should understand that even tiny amounts of cheating can spoil the overall effect of the diet, and that their friendship, support, and encouragement are crucial to its success.

THE INTERNET

The Internet is an increasingly common source of information and support for parents of children with health problems, including epilepsy. The feedback we receive from parents who use the Internet to obtain information about the ketogenic diet indicates that this information is of greatly varying quality:

- Some of the information is excellent and very valuable.
- Some of the information is incorrect and/or misleading.
- Some of the information shows the bias of an enthusiastic parent.
- Some of the information shows the bias of a disgruntled parent.

If you use or intend to use the Internet as a source of information on the ketogenic diet, be aware of the varying quality of information you may be receiving. Keep in mind the source of the information. The challenge is to separate the useful information on the ketogenic diet from that which is incorrect.

EVERYTHING WENT REALLY WELL FOR US. *We were really careful, read every label, and never gave her anything that wasn't allowed. We followed the rules to the nth degree. And she never had any more seizures.*

—MH

CHAPTER ELEVEN

GOING OFF THE DIET

Children who get good benefit from the ketogenic diet traditionally remain on the 4:1 ketogenic ratio for 2 years or until they have been seizure-free without medication for 1 full year. Then they switch to a 3:1 diet ratio for 6 months. If they remain seizure-free, this is followed by a 2:1 ratio for 6 months, after which they are weaned off the diet and can eat any foods they want.

The above schedule is somewhat arbitrary, and no studies have been performed yet to detail the best way for discontinuing the diet. The 2-year time figure is the result of tradition rather than science, although studies of diet discontinuation are in progress.

Approximately 29 percent of children who start on the diet discontinue it within 6 months of initiation, most because the diet is ineffective or too difficult. If the family and ketoteam determine that the ketogenic diet is not the best therapy for a child, the discontinuation can be taken more rapidly, normally over a period of weeks. If a serious medical problem or other special situation arises, the ketoteam will determine the most effective way of discontinuing the diet. In all cases, discontinuation of the diet should be carried out under the guidance of a trained ketoteam—a knowledgeable physician, a trained nurse, or an experienced dietician.

This traditional regimen for easing off the diet over the course of a year may be more cautious than is absolutely necessary, but we believe it is better to err on the side of caution. There has been concern (although without much evidence) that withdrawing too abruptly from the diet could bring back seizures, and possibly even status epilepticus, wiping out all those months of discipline. We have not seen this happen.

The length of time a child has to stay on the 4:1 ratio is sometimes extended by a year or two if a child has not stuck to the regimen strictly or if some other reason exists to think more time on the diet will help the child. The child who has had a good, but incomplete response to the diet, and for whom the diet is not a burden, may continue the diet. We have had children who have remained on the diet as long as 11 years. For some children whose seizures have not been completely controlled, it is possible to continue the diet beyond 2 years to maintain the degree of control that has been achieved.

Clearly, the diet does not have to be discontinued after 2 years, but this duration gives the child and the family some light at the end of the tunnel when they are first embarking on the diet. Future research may indicate that the diet may be discontinued after a shorter time, but, at present, we continue it for 2 years.

No research has indicated any chemical or metabolic reason for stopping the diet after 2 successful years rather than staying on it longer; it is just good for the child and the family to get back to a normal life.

The question of when to discontinue the diet is particularly urgent for the many children whose seizures are 50 percent to 90 percent or more improved, but who are not made seizure-free by the diet. Will their seizures increase after discontinuation? Will medications have to be reinstituted? These questions remain to be studied. Continuing the diet in this case is an alternative to the increased medications that will/may be needed if the diet is stopped. If a child has an increase in her seizures, or begins to have seizures again once the diet has ended (this is very rare), it is possible to restart the diet.

BEN HAS BEEN ON THE DIET FOR 9 YEARS NOW. *He is severely retarded and fed by gastrostomy. His cholesterol is 116. He has had no seizures in more than 8 years. Taper the diet? Why would we do that? The diet is no trouble for us and makes no difference to Ben.*

—TM

The long-term consequences of remaining on the ketogenic diet for many years have been recently studied, and most children do very well. Some handicapped children have been maintained on the diet for 6 to 11 years without obvious ill effects. The risk of kidney stones and fractures is about 1 in 4, so this must be closely watched, but no child had very significantly elevated cholesterol levels (above 400). Studies have shown that lipids and triglycerides are elevated during the diet to levels that would normally be considered to increase the threat of stroke or heart disease after a lifetime of exposure. The potential threat of stroke or heart disease after a limited exposure of 2 or even 10 years of a high-fat diet has not been studied. Any health threat would have to be evaluated in relation to alternative health risks posed by uncontrolled epilepsy, such as increased seizures or increased long-term intake of anticonvulsant medications.

I HAD NOT SEEN OR HEARD FROM TYLER in many years when his family the clinic. Tyler was now a late teenager, with cerebral palsy and moderate called to ask if they could increase his calories. We asked them to come to retardation. He had been on the diet for 15 years. He had grown and was doing well, but still had one or two seizures per year. He was on no medications, and the family did not want to use any. "He's doing just fine on the diet," they said. "We just want him to gain a bit of weight."

—JMF

This case also provides an example of why we try to see the patients once a year, even if they are doing "just fine."

THE QUICK-DISCONTINUATION METHOD

The decision of when to come off the diet is, for the most part, left to the parents. Some, especially those for whom the diet's benefits are not dramatic, wonder early on whether the diet is worth the trouble. They want to know what the difference would be if their child was on a normal diet. For these parents, we sometimes suggest a relatively quick test of the diet:

Continue the diet, but substitute whole milk for the heavy cream over a 2-week trial period. This is roughly equivalent to switching from a 4:1 diet to a 3:1 ketogenic ratio and is easy to undo if seizures occur because it does not disrupt the diet's ritual. (Going off the diet entirely for 2 weeks, on the other hand, may permanently alter the child's or family's willingness to comply with the diet's rigors.)

If no change occurs in seizure activity during the following week or two, then substitute skim milk for the whole milk. This is approximately the equivalent of going to a 2:1 ketogenic ratio.

If seizure activity does not change over the next week or so on the lower ratio, then the family often chooses to discontinue the diet entirely.

Although we have not assessed this plan in a rigorous fashion, it may provide a useful alternative to recalculating meal plans in order to let a borderline family test discontinuation of the diet.

DEBORAH RETURNED FOR HER 3-MONTH FOLLOW-UP VISIT. *While the diet had substantially reduced her seizures and had allowed her to stop one of her medications, both Deborah and her mother were finding it very difficult. They wanted to discontinue the diet. We suggested testing the diet's effectiveness using our "quick method," substituting whole milk for the cream for a 2-week trial. After only 1 week, Deborah's mother called to ask if she could switch back to cream, because Deborah's seizures had grown much worse since switching to milk.*

—JMF

Some children who have responded exceptionally well to the diet start to come off it before the 2-year mark is reached. This decision is often suggested by the parents and agreed to in consultation with the physicians.

Toward the end, we started letting him smell things. The other kids would give him a sniff of what they were eating, and he would say, "I can have that when I'm off the diet, right?"

—CC

SHE WAS A JUNIOR BRIDESMAID at a wedding the day she went off the diet. That was when she was 12. We had checked with Mrs. Kelly and agreed to let her eat cake at the reception. All of us were very apprehensive. There had been a lot of anxiety each time we cut the ratio, but she kept doing well, so sweets were the last test. Nobody else at the reception really knew what we were going through—it was a private thing among us and our very close friends. When she ate the cake and had no problems, it was thrilling for us. After that we were probably cautious for another week or two. Now, she won't look at whipped cream, but she eats just like a typical teenager—pizza and candy and all the typical teenage food.

—MH

WE HAD BEEN DOWN TO A 1:1 RATIO FOR A FEW MONTHS *when one day the doctor said, "Why don't you take him out for an ice cream sundae—you're off the diet!" Well, I couldn't quite do that, but we did take him for a steak and potato dinner. Then, about an hour later, I got him a little dish of mint chocolate chip ice cream. It was very dramatic for me to see him eat a real meal. And for him, too—his little eyes were watering. It was a tear-jerking experience. We had finally made it! He used to be an extremely picky eater but now he just really enjoys eating.*

—JS

AFTER HE HAD DONE PERFECTLY FOR A YEAR AND A HALF *on the 4:1 diet, we had done 6 months on the 3:1, and then a couple of months on the 2:1, when his sixth birthday was coming up. We asked him what he wanted, and he said pizza. Well, you're nervous as can be, but he was doing so well that we decided to stop the diet on* *his birthday, before the full 6 months of the 2:1 were up. We invited all the neighborhood kids in, and I put candles in the pizza. After he took the first bite, he looked up at me and said, "Dad, this is the best birthday present I've ever had."*

—RZ

ANXIETY AND RELIEF

It is natural for a parent to feel anxious when a child is going off the diet. After all that time spent planning and measuring food to the accuracy of a gram, it's hard to kick the habit! All we can tell nervous parents is that ending the diet is to their child's advantage once the child is seizure-free for 2 years. The ketogenic diet therapy's goal is to treat a problem—seizures. Once the problem is gone, the therapy should also end.

A child can start going off the diet once the full benefits of the diet have been realized. Exactly when this invisible finish line has been crossed will vary for each child. But by the time a child has been on the diet rigidly for 2 years and is seizure-free, its long-term benefits will most likely have already been gained. If the EEG has returned to normal, for example, it is likely to stay normal. Even if the EEG is still abnormal, it may be possible for the child who has been seizure-free for 2 years to go off the diet gradually without the return of seizures. The child is likely to remain seizure-free when normal eating is resumed if no seizures have occurred with no medication during the diet.

__AFTER WE HAD BEEN ON THE 2:1 DIET FOR ABOUT 6 WEEKS,__ I asked what was next, and Mrs. Kelly said I could give him some popcorn with lots of butter. I was so nervous I was shaking when I gave it to him. He felt the same way. "Are you sure she said I could have popcorn?" he asked me. I almost didn't know how to gradually withdraw the diet. When it came time to go off it, the thought of giving him a glass of low-fat milk *instead of cream made me crazy with nerves.*

—CC

***GOING OFF THE DIET WAS VERY LIBERATING.** At last, we could go places without planning and thinking about every meal. We could spend a day at the mall. She could go to parties and eat what the other kids were having. It was great.*

—MH

Meals with lower ketogenic ratios are increasingly similar to regular meals. A 2:1 ratio will seem almost like a normal diet, compared with the 4:1 meals. There will be room for a lot more meat and vegetables and even the possibility of some carbohydrates.

Once a child has been weaned down to a 2:1 ratio, and has been on that ratio for a few months, we recommend that formerly forbidden foods be gradually introduced into the diet. We encourage parents to start with somewhat fatty foods, such as buttery popcorn, greasy french fries, and hamburgers. Sometimes we go to a 1:1 ratio for a few months, which can be useful as a tapering method, even though at this ratio the child is no longer in ketosis. In general, though, when the gradually introduced foods have reached a point where the child is no longer in ketosis, you're home free!

FOR ME, THE DIET REALLY WASN'T ALL THAT HARD. *There wasn't a single day when I resented having to weigh the meals. For me it was a very pleasant experience. It was just a miracle.*

—JS

SECTION III
CALCULATIONS

CHAPTER TWELVE

CALCULATING THE KETOGENIC DIET

The initial calculation of the ketogenic diet is three parts science and one part art. It requires a full nutritional assessment and an understanding of the child's medical condition. The art is a combination of experience, prioritization, empathy, and intuition. In each case, a child's individual needs must be taken into account.

ESTIMATING CALORIC NEEDS

Calculating the caloric requirements of an individual child requires consideration of both the child's current and desirable weight, as well as her activity level. The estimated caloric needs for infants and children, as published in *The Nutrition Manual for At-risk Infants and Toddlers,* is shown in Table 12-1.

NOTE: These estimates are for children with average activity levels. They may be too high for profoundly impaired children and those with impaired activity levels.

TABLE12-1: Estimating Calorie Needs for Infants and Children

Age (yr)	BMR (kcal/kg)	SDA+EXC (kcal/kg)	Activity (kcal/kg)	Growth (kcal/kg)	Total (kcal/kg)
0–0.5	55	20	17	20	112
0.5–1	55	17	20	13	105
1–2	40	17	22	11	90
3–4	40	14	21	10	85

BMR=Basal metabolic rate, which is similar to REE+< 10%; it ispercent; this componentof energy expenditure that is increased during fever or other stress

SDA=Specific dynamic action or energy required for digestion and absorption

EXC=Energy lost through excretion

Reference: Reprinted with permission from Lowrey. Growth and Development in Children,6th ed. Chicago: Year Book, 1973

Source: The Nutrition Manual for At-risk Infants and Toddlers. Precept Press, 1992, p.231.

Children's energy requirements vary greatly, depending on activity levels, stage of growth phase, and individual constitution. It is usually recommended that ideal weight for length or height ("expected" weight for length or height, or 50th percentile weight for length or height) be used to calculate caloric needs. However, if muscle mass is lower or higher than normal, estimated "lean body weight" may be used.

As indicated in Table 12-1, the basal metabolic rate for a child 1 to 2 years of age is 40kcal/kg. Then 17kcal/kg are added for specific dynamic action, 22kcal for activity, and 11kcal for growth. The caloric requirement for an *average* 1-to 2-year-old child is therefore 90kcal/kg (40+17+22+11=90).

The ketogenic diet is generally based on 85 percent of Recommended Daily Allowance (RDA) of calories for a child's desirable weight and height, but it can be modified to allow for such factors as the child's activity level, natural rate of metabolism, and local climate.

The goal of the diet is to provide optimal seizure control and maintain adequate nutrition for growth. When we make our initial estimates of a child's dietary needs, we begin by assessing the age, weight, height, health, activity status, and a current 3-day food record for each child. The ketogenic diet appears to work best when the child is neither too fat nor too lean, when she is close to her "desirable body weight" and body mass index (BMI) for age. This is defined as the 50th percentile of weight for height.

Underweight children must gain weight in order to have sufficient fat reserves to burn between meals. Overweight children need to lose weight, because if too much body fat is present, a child may have difficulty obtaining sufficient ketosis to control seizures. Severely handicapped children may be smaller in size and weight than average for their age. As a rule, when initiating the ketogenic diet, we use desirable (50th percentile) weight for height in estimating a child's caloric needs on the ketogenic diet.

That is just the start, however, since the child's activity level is also an important determinant of her caloric needs. A very active child needs more calories than a less active one. Profoundly handicapped children, who sometimes are very inactive, usually require fewer calories per kilogram than an average child. A diet calculated for desirable body weight in a child of average mobility may cause a profoundly handicapped child to gain weight, and it will not provide sufficient ketosis.

Providing approximately 85 percent of the calories normally recommended for the child's age and desirable weight should be enough to allow most children to grow normally and remain close to their desirable weight for their age and height. We continually monitor for disproportionate weight gain or loss throughout the time on the diet. Obtaining a diet/food record prior to the ketogenic diet initiation is essential in estimating individual energy needs.

PROTEIN

Recommended daily protein allowances are calculated for average children of a given height and weight and an average activity level. The ketogenic diet, however, is rarely used for average children. Striving to reach an RDA of protein as close to the normal for age is important. In adolescents, it may be difficult to achieve the proper fat to carbohydrate ratio if 1g of protein per kilo of body weight is given. In this case, we may use as little as 0.75g of protein per kilogram. We use U.S. government's RDA and World Health Organization standards as guidelines (Table 12-2). Growth is closely monitored every 3 to 6 months, and is used as a guide for adequate nutrition.

The most important factor in the successful and safe initiation of the diet is close contact between the family and the ketogenic diet team during the early weeks. Given that a detailed nutritional assessment and lab work are essential to the initial diet prescription, four main areas exist to which the physician's and dietitian's judgment must be applied in determining the input values for the ketogenic diet calculation:

TABLE 12-2: Protein Allowances

Age	RDA for Protein (g/kg)	WHO Mean Protein Allowance (g/kg)
0–6 months	2.2	1.38
6–12 months	1.6	1.21
1–3 years	1.2	0.97
4–6 years	1.1	0.84
7–10 years	1.0	0.8
Males 11–14 yrs	1.0	0.79
Males 15–18 yrs	0.9	0.69
Females 11–14 yrs	1.0	0.76
Females 15–18 yrs	0.8	0.64
Adults	0.8	—

Reproduced with permission from Recommended Dietary Allowances, 10th edition. Wash-ington, DC: National Academy Press, 1989.

- Desirable weight versus actual weight
- Calories per kilogram
- Ketogenic ratio (fat: (protein+carbohydrate))
- Fluid allotment

DESIRABLE WEIGHT VERSUS ACTUAL WEIGHT

Although the diet traditionally approximated 85 percent of RDAs, individualized caloric values based on current versus desirable weight, activity levels, and a food record of current intake will provide better nutrition.

The initial ketogenic ratio is usually 4:1, unless a child is very young, very overweight, or has a very fragile medical condition. In the case of a very overweight child, the 3:1 diet will be based on a desirable weight that is lower than the current weight, and this should lead to some weight loss.

In the case of a child who is substantially underweight, a dietitian may want to base the child's calories/kilogram on the current weight and then slowly increase the calories by small increments. A child with feeding problems or recurrent aspiration may benefit from a feeding tube or gastrostomy before starting the diet. If the diet is very effective, though, eating ability and activity levels may improve, and calories may need to be raised.

Children on the diet should be weighed every week, and the weights written down by the parents or recorded on a growth chart. Weights should be taken at the same time of day, prior to a meal, and without clothes. If excess weight gain occurs, the child is receiving too many calories. If excess weight loss occurs, the calories may need to be increased. Over the longer term, children should gain weight in proportion to their growth in height. Children should be measured every 3 months in their physician's office, their height and weight plotted on a growth chart, and calories should be adjusted to keep weight proportional to growth.

FLUID ALLOTMENT

Although fluid restriction has not been well studied, and its importance to the diet is not entirely clear, anecdotal evidence indicates that fluid intake levels may affect seizure control in children on the ketogenic diet. Fluid allotments are set at about 85 to 100 percent of maintenance for healthy, active children (see Chapter 7):

BODY WEIGHT	FLUID ALLOTMENT
1–10kg	100mLl/kg
10–20kg	1,000mL+50mL/kg for each kg < 10kg
<20kg	1,500mL+20mL/kg for eachkg < 20kg

Fluid allocation should be individualized and increased with an increase in activity or a hot climate. Fluids are not restricted during illness, and are increased to 100mL/kg for fragile children and infants less than 1 year of age.

Urine specific gravity should be 1.010 to 1.025, and should be used as a guide to adequate hydration.

JAMES: A CASE STUDY

Designing a diet for a fictitious child called James illustrates the thought process of a dietitian evaluating an individual coming in for ketogenic diet initiation:

Background/History

James is a 4-year-7-month-old male with history of infantile spasms (myoclonic seizures) and developmental delay. Seizure onset was at 12 months of age. Seizure frequency is 100 to 150 jerks per day, and he has occasional generalized tonic-clonic seizures.

James's current medications are Topamax 75mg BID, Depakote 375mg TID, and Tranxene 0.9mg daily. He also takes Bugs Bunny multivitamin/mineral supplements.

No current laboratory test values are available for James.

James feeds himself. He has no problems with chewing or swallowing, and he has no history of pneumonia or aspiration.

James's mother reports his appetite to be poor and states that he is a "picky eater." James normally eats a great deal of starches (pasta, bread, etc.) as well as vegetables. He does not like meat very much. He eats three meals and two snacks daily. His food preferences have been recorded.

His activity is low to normal—James takes soccer once a week and participates in recess at pre-school. His bowel movements are normal for the most part. He has no known food allergies or intolerances.

Three-day food recall

James's average intake is 1,290kcal, 42gm protein, with a vitamin/mineral consumption that is adequate, with the exception of calcium.

Weight and height

James weight and height record is:
- WT: 18.4kg, Ht 111.8cm (40.5lbs, 44 inches)
- WT FOR AGE: 50–75%
- HT FOR AGE: 75–90%
- WT FOR HT: 25–50%

His ideal body weight is 19.4kg (wt for ht at 50 percent), so James is presently at 95 percent of his ideal body weight.

James's growth pattern has been relatively normal—both height and weight were proportional, following the 75 percent to 90 percent curve until 6 months ago. His mother said that James has been the same weight for 6 months now, despite an increase in height. She attributes his lack of weight gain to a decreased appetite since the addition of Topamax.

Physical assessment

No physical signs of deficiencies are present; James appears to be well nourished, although quite lean.

Assessment

James does not appear to be at nutritional risk at this point. Despite not gaining weight for 6 months, he is still 95 percent of his ideal weight, and his weight has crossed only one percentile. He looks healthy, is consuming what is recommended for his age in the way of protein and macro-and micronutrients (with the exception of a calcium intake of only 700mg). His caloric intake is obviously too low, as seen by the lack of weight gain and the fact that James is under his ideal body weight. It is reasonable to start him at his current caloric intake at a 4:1 ratio. We do not want him to lose weight, and the high ratio will allow us to provide the fat needed for ketosis via the diet.

Initial Diet

James initial diet was calculated to contain the following values:

- 1,300kcal, 4:1 ratio, 1,200cc total fluid daily. To be given in three equal meals and a snack of 150kcal before bedtime.
- kcal: 1,300 (70.7kcal/kg body weight)
- Total protein: 24.5gm (1.3gm/kg ideal body weight)
- Total carbohydrate: 8gm
- Total fat: 130gm
- Total fluid: 1,200cc (80 percent of estimated maintenance needs)

Goals

The stated goals of James's diet are:

- Seizure control.
- Attaining ideal weight within 3-month period. Increasing his kcal intake in small increments (5 to 10 percent of kcal every 2 to 4 weeks) should be sufficient to attain this

goal, provided that seizures are well controlled. James will probably not only have an improved appetite, but hopefully improved activity as well, if his seizures can be controlled.

- Maintaining optimal nutritional status (maintaining growth and overall nutritional status long term).
- Weaning medications once the diet is fine-tuned satisfactorily.

Plan

The plan for James's initiation of the diet involves a step-by-step process:

1. Implement diet, educate parents.
2. Attain biochemical indices to check nutritional status (visceral protein status, anemias, electrolytes, hydration, renal function, etc.).
3. Discuss Topamax wean with physicians. Weaning this medication aggressively might help improve James's appetite.
4. Order multivitamin/mineral supplement that meets patient's recommended micronutrient needs 100 percent.

5.   Continue to track height, weight, seizure control, etc. via phone/e-mail/fax.
6.   See James at 3-month follow-up visit.

GENERAL RULES FOR INITIAL KETOGENIC DIET CALCULATION

Once judgments are made about James's ideal weight, ketogenic ratio, and liquid allotment, the ketogenic diet can be calculated. Although computer software makes calculating the menus much faster and easier, it is useful to understand the steps of the calculation so that it can be modified, if necessary, to meet a child's individual needs:

1.   Decide on an optimal level of calories. This should be done using a thorough medical and nutritional history and the dietitian and physician's professional judgment. Variables such as the child's activity level, frame size, medical condition, and recent

weight gain or loss must be taken into account.

2. Set the desired ketogenic ratio. Most children are started on a 4:1 ketogenic ratio. Very overweight or medically compromised children may be started on a 3:1 or 3.5:1 ratio of fat and protein to carbohydrates. Children under 2 years of age and adolescents are usually started on a 3:1 ratio.

3. Liquid levels should be set at about 85 to 100 percent of maintenance for healthy, active children. Liquids are increased for fragile children and infants under 1 year of age. Urine specific gravity should be used as a guide to adequate hydration.

4. Always strive to attain RDAs for protein (and never allow protein to fall below World Health Organization standards).

5. The ketogenic diet must be supplemented *daily* with calcium and a carbohydrate-free multivitamin with minerals. The diet is not nutritionally sufficient without supplementation.

Because this book is written for both parents and medical professionals, and because we believe that the diet works best with informed parents as part of the team, we believe it is important to know as much about the diet as possible.

> **NOTE:** The ketogenic diet should *never* be attempted without careful medical and nutritional supervision.

ROSEANNE IS A GIRL WHO ALMOST DIED because her parents started her on the ketogenic diet without consulting a doctor. She was 5 years old when she was admitted to Hopkins' intensive care unit with pneumonia, dehydration, and a very low pulse rate. There were major concerns about whether she would survive the night. She appeared wasted, cachectic, and looked as though she had been starved by her parents.

The nurse called the child abuse team. The parents arrived a few minutes later, having followed the ambulance from the referring hospital. They seemed very nice and very concerned. They said that Roseanne had suffered from lack of oxygen at birth and was quite developmentally delayed. At 5 years, she still could not sit by herself or communicate. Roseanne had experienced seizures since she was 6 months old and had been treated with many medications, but without much success. Her parents had come to the conclusion that not only were the medications not helping, but their side effects were part of the reason for Roseanne's lack of progress.

"All those doctors were doing was experimenting on our daughter," they said.

Then the parents had seen Jim Abrams' TV movie about a diet for epilepsy that would "get you off the medications." When they called Hopkins, they were told that Hopkins would not be able to admit Roseanne for the diet for several months. Her parents felt they couldn't wait that long, so they started the diet by themselves.

"It wasn't so hard at first," they said, and the seizures were better, until the last month when she just didn't seem to want to eat. Then she started throwing up and breathing funny. "I guess now you'll have to admit her!" the parents said.

Roseanne had pneumonia, but was also severely acidotic, malnourished, and dehydrated. With intensive care, over the course of a week, she gradually came around and was able to be discharged home, but not on the diet. Until she had built up her reserves and had become better nourished, we felt that the diet posed too much of a risk. Frustration with the medical profession and impatience with the processes involved almost resulted in the child's death.

How a dietitian calculates the diet: an example

1. **AGE AND WEIGHT.** Fill out the following information:
    Age _____

Desirable weight in kilograms
___

Mary has been prescribed a 4:1 ketogenic diet. She is 4 years old and currently weighs 15 kilograms (33 pounds). Her dietitian has determined that this weight is appropriate for Mary.

2. **CALORIES PER KILOGRAM.** After a full medical and nutritional assessment, a dietitian will assign a calorie per kilogram level for diet initiation.

The dietitian has set Mary's diet at 72kcal/kg. (Note that this figure involves a dietitian's judgment; it is slightly higher than 85 percent of caloric needs if estimated from Table 12-1 (85kcal/kgx.85=72kcal/kg).

3. **TOTAL CALORIES.** Determine the total number of calories in the diet by multiplying the child's weight by the number of calories set per kilogram.

Mary, age 4 and weighing 15 kilograms, needs a total of 72x15 or 1,085 calories per day.

4. **DIETARY UNIT COMPOSITION.**
Dietary units are the building blocks of the ketogenic diet. A 4:1 diet has dietary units made up of 4g of fat to each 1g of protein and 1g of carbohydrate. Because fat has 9 calories perg (9x4=36), and protein and carbohydrate each have 4 calories perg (4x1=4), a dietary unit at a 4:1 diet ratio has 36+4=40 calories. The caloric value and breakdown of dietary units vary with the ketogenic ratio:

RATIO	FAT CALORIES	CARBOHYDRATE PLUS PROTEIN CALORIES	CALORIES PER DIETARY UNIT
2:1	2gx9kcal/g=18	1gx4kcal/g=4	18+4=22
3:1	3gx9kcal/g=27	1gx4kcal/g=4	27+4=31
4:1	4gx9kcal/g=36	1gx4kcal/g=4	36+4=40
5:1	5gx9kcal/g=45	1gx4kcal/g=4	45+4=49

Mary's dietary units will be made up of 40 calories each, because she is on a 4:1 ratio.

5. **DIETARY UNIT QUANTITY.**
Divide the total calories allotted (Step 3) by the number of

calories in each dietary unit (Step 4) to determine the number of dietary units to be allowed daily.

Each of Mary's dietary units on a 4:1 ratio contains 40 calories, and she is allowed a total of 1,085kcal/day, so she gets 1,085/40=27 dietary units per day.

6. **FAT ALLOWANCE.** Multiply the number of dietary units by the units of fat in the prescribed ketogenic ratio to determine theg of fat permitted daily.

On her 4:1 diet, with 27 dietary units/day, Mary will have 27x4 or 108g of fat per day.

7. **PROTEIN+CARBOHYDRATE ALLOWANCE.** Multiply the number of dietary units by the number of units of protein+carbohydrate in the prescribed ketogenic ratio, usually one, to determine the c o m b i n e d   d a i l y protein+carbohydrate allotment.

On her 4:1 diet, Mary will have 27x1 or 27g of protein and carbohydrate per day.

8. **PROTEIN ALLOWANCE.** The dietitian will determine optimal

protein levels as part of the nutritional assessment, taking into account such factors as age, growth, activity level, and medical condition.

Mary's dietitian has determined that she needs 1.2g of protein per kilogram of body weight (18g total).

9. **CARBOHYDRATE ALLOWANCE.** Determine carbohydrate allowance by subtracting protein from the total carbohydrate+protein allowance (Step 7 minus Step 8). Carbohydrates are the diet's filler and are always determined last.

Mary's carbohydrate allowance is 27-18=9g of carbohydrate daily.

10. **MEAL ORDER.** Divide the daily fat, protein, and carbohydrate allotments into the desired number of meals and snacks per day. The number of meals will be based on the child's dietary habits and nutritional needs. It is essential that the proper ratio of fat: protein+carbohydrate be maintained at each meal.

Mary's dietitian has decided to give her three meals and no snacks per day:

	DAILY	PER MEAL
Protein	18 g	6 g
Fat	108.0 g	36.0 g
Carbohydrate	9 g	3.0 g
Calories	1,085	361

Note: This example is simplified for teaching purposes. In reality most 4-year-olds would be prescribed one or two snacks in addition to their three meals. The snacks would be in the same ratio (4:1), and the meals reduced by the number of calories in each snack.

11. **LIQUIDS.** Multiply the child's desirable weight by the value shown on the chart listed earlier in this chapter to determine the daily allotment of liquid. Liquid intake should be spaced throughout the day. Liquids should be noncaloric, such as water or decaffeinated zero-calorie diet drinks. In hot

climates, the cream may be excluded from the fluid allowance (in other words, liquids may be increased by the volume of the cream in the diet). The liquid allotment may also be set equal to the number of calories in the diet.

Mary, who weighs 15kg, is allowed 1,000+(50x5)=1,250mLx.9=1,125cc of fluid per day, including her allotted cream.

12.   **DIETARY SUPPLEMENTS.** The ketogenic diet is deficient in some nutrients. Multivitamin and mineral supplements are required. When choosing a supplement, it is important to consider carbohydrate content. Children who are not medically compromised can usually be adequately supplemented with an over-the-counter, reputable multivitamin and mineral supplement and a separate calcium supplement. Unicap, Centrum, and Poly-Vi-Sol have been used in the past, although

the composition of branded products is always subject to change. Most children do well with commercially available supplements, although these have been alleged to lack some micronutrients.

CALCULATING MEAL PLANS

Calculating the meal plans themselves, in contrast to the diet prescription, is a fairly straightforward procedure. Currently, two different ways are used to calculate the meal plans: by hand or by computer.

The hand calculation method uses exchange lists and rounded nutritional values for simplicity. This method is cumbersome, time-consuming, and based to a certain extent on nutritional averages. It is, however, the method used at Johns Hopkins and elsewhere with much success before the availability of personal computers. It is important that dietitians become familiar with the hand calculation method in order to fully understand the logic of meal planning, and in case a computer is not available in a pinch.

Several computer programs are available at many centers and these are used by the dietitian to create meal plans. Because the computer program uses data about the precise nutritional content of specific foods, whereas the hand calculation method relies on averages in order to simplify the math, the computer program may result in slightly different numbers of calories and g for a given meal than the hand calculation method.

No program should be initiated or changed without the oversight of a dietitian to be certain that the nutritional information is up-to-date. Generic Group A and B vegetables and fruits can be exchanged with both methods of meal calculation. It is easy for parents to switch from one Group A vegetable to another, or one 10 percent fruit to another, depending on the child's whims or what is available in the grocery store. The exchange lists assume that some variety in the diet will be present. If the child only likes carrots and grapes—which contain the highest carbohydrate levels on the exchange lists—then she could end up with less than optimal seizure control. In this case, the meal plans should be recalculated specifically for carrots and grapes.

The precision of the computer calculations shows the minor differences between the content of, say, broccoli and green beans. For most children, these minor differences are of little importance. Therefore, once the computer has calculated a meal plan, and assuming that the child is doing well on the diet, exchanges may still be made among the foods on the fruit and vegetable exchange lists. If better seizure control is needed, however, it may in some cases be achieved through the use of specific meal-plan calculations instead of exchange lists.

With the availability of the computer program, we no longer use meat exchange lists. Meats' fat and carbohydrate contents vary too greatly. The exchange lists are still used with hand calculations.

The dietitian provides parents with a set of basic meal plans before they go home from the hospital. When parents call the dietitian to discuss meal plans, they can refer to these basic meals by title. The basic meal plans are:

1. Meat/fish/poultry, fruit/vegetable, fat, cream.
2. Cheese, fruit/vegetable, fat, cream.
3. Egg, fruit/vegetable, fat, cream.

The meat and cheese should be designated specifically (i.e., chicken, fish, Parmesan) in actual meal plans. When specifics are added, the result will probably be a basic set of six or eight meal plans sent home with the parents from the hospital.

AVERAGE FOOD VALUES FOR HAND CALCULATIONS

	Grams	Protein	Carb.	Fat
36% Cream	100	2.0	36.0	3.0
Ground Beef	100	24.2	19.1	—
Chicken	100	31.1	2.6	0
Tuna in Water	100	26.8	1.8	0
10% Fruit	100	1.0	0.0	10
Group B Vegetable	100	2.0	0.0	7.0

Fat	100	0.0	74.0	—
Egg	100	12.0	12.0	—
Cheese	100	30.0	35.3	—
Cottage Cheese (4%)	100	13.2	4.4	3.5
Cream Cheese	100	6.7	33.3	3.3
Peanut Butter	100	26.0	48.0	22.0

Note: A food contents reference book, such as Bowes & Church'sFood Values, is helpful for current information on specific foods. Asdiscussed in Chapter 5, the fat content of heavy cream should be con-sistent (e.g., 36 percent), and butter should come in solid, stick form, not whipped or low calorie.

CROSS MULTIPLICATION: THE KEY TO USING THE FOOD LIST

Question: If 100g of 36 percent cream contains 3.0g carbohydrate, how much cream contains 2.4g of carbohydrate?

$$\text{Step 1:} \quad \frac{100}{3} = \frac{x}{2.4}$$

$$\text{Step 2:} \quad 3x = 240$$

Step 3: $\quad x = \dfrac{240}{3} = 80\,g$

Answer: 80g of 36% cream contains 2.4g of carbohydrate.

Sample calculation

1. Jeremy, a 9-year-3-month-old boy, is to be placed on a 4:1 ketogenic diet. His actual weight is 32kg and his height is 134cm. According to the standard charts, he is at 50 percent for height but 90 percent for weight. His ideal weight is estimated at 29kg.
2. The dietitian estimated Jeremy's calorie allotment at 60 calories per kilogram. One of the dietitian's goals was to have Jeremy gradually achieve his ideal weight. Toward this end, Jeremy's total calorie allotment is set by multiplying his ideal weight by 60: 29x60=1,740 calories per day.
3. Each of Jeremy's dietary units will consist of 4g fat (9 calories per g)=36 calories 1g carbohydrate+protein (4 calories

per g)=4 calories Total calories per dietary unit=40 calories

4. Jeremy's dietary units will be determined by dividing his total daily calorie allotment (Step 2) by the calories in each dietary unit: 1,740 calories/40 calories per dietary unit=43.5 dietary units per day.

5. Jeremy's daily fat allowance is determined by multiplying his dietary units (Step 4 above) by the fat component in his diet ratio (4 in a 4:1 ratio):43.5x4=174g fat.

6. Jeremy's protein needs are at a minimum 1g of protein per kilogram of body weight. His ideal weight is 29kg, so he needs at least 29.0g protein daily.

7. Jeremy's daily carbohydrate allotment is determined by multiplying his dietary units (Step 4 above) by the 1 in his 4:1 ratio, then subtracting his necessary protein (Step 6 above) from the total: 43.5-29=14.5g carbohydrate per day.

Jeremy's complete diet order will read:

	PER DAY	PER MEAL
Protein	29.0 g	9.7 g
Fat	174.0 g	58.0 g
Carbohydrate	14.5 g	4.8 g
Calories	1,740	580

Note: Most children are now given a meal plan that includes one or two snacks, which would diminish the quantity of food in the three-main meals. If Jeremy does not lose weight, is not in sufficient ketosis, or turns out to not be as active as originally thought, the caloricamounts will be recalculated during the fine-tuning period.

CALCULATING A MEAL	JEREMY'S TUNA SALAD
1. Calculate the whipping cream first. Heavy whipping cream should take up no more than half of the carbohydrate allotment in a meal.	1. Jeremy is allowed a total of 4.8g carbohydrate per meal. To use half of this carbohydrate allotment as cream, calculate the amount of 36 percent cream that contains 2.4g of carbohydrate. (See note on cross-multiplication.) Jeremy should eat 80g of 36 percent cream, which contains 2.4g of carbohydrate.
2. Calculate the rest of the carbohydrates (fruit or vegetables) by subtracting the carbohydrate contained in the cream from the total carbohydrate allotment.	2. For his remaining 2.4g of carbohydrate, Jeremy can eat 35g of Group B vegetables, or twice as many Group A vegetables.

3. Calculate the remaining protein (chicken, cheese, or egg) by subtracting the protein in the cream and vegetables from the total protein allowance. The total amount of protein may occasionally be off by 0.1g (over or under) without adverse effect.

3. The 34.3g Group B vegetables and 80g 36 percent cream contain a total of 2.3g protein (0.68 _1.6 _ 2.3). Jeremy is allowed 9.7g protein per meal, so he can eat as much tuna as contains 9.7–2.3 _ 7.4g protein. Referring to the food values chart, this works out to be 28g tuna.

4. Calculate the amount of fat to be allowed in the meal by subtracting the fat in the cream and protein from the total fat allowance.

4. Jeremy has to eat 58g fat with each meal. The cream and tuna contain 29.3g fat, leaving 28.7g of fat to be mixed in with his tuna fish. Jeremy will get 39g mayonnaise, which contains 28.9g fat. (Note that mayonnaise actually has fewer g of fat than oil does and also contains some protein and carbohydrate. The hand calculation method does not account for these variations.)

CALCULATING MEAL PLAN

	Weight	Protein	Fat	Carbohydrate
Tuna	28 g	7.4 g	0.5 g	—
Group B Vegetable	33 g	0.7 g	—	2.3
Fat	39 g	—	28.9 g	—

36% Cream	80 g	1.6 g	28.8 g	2.4 g
Actual To-tal		9.7 g	58.2 g	4.7 g
Should Be		9.7 g	58.0 g	4.8 g

The 4:1 ketogenic ratio of this menu may be double-checked by adding the grams of protein □ carbohydrate in the meal and multiplying by 4. The result should be the amount of fat in the meal, in this case 58 g. Since (9.7+4.8)x4=58, the ratio is correct.

NOTES ON JEREMY'S LUNCH

- Jeremy likes his cream frozen in an ice cream ball (slightly whipped), flavored with vanilla and saccharin, and sprinkled with a little cinnamon.
- Jeremy's mom arranges the vegetables in thin-sliced crescents or shoestring sticks around the tuna.
- If Jeremy doesn't like as much mayonnaise with his tuna, some of his fat allowance in the form of oil can be calculated and whipped into the cream one hour after it goes into the freezer. The fats on the

exchange list can be used interchangeably—a meal's fat can be provided as all mayonnaise, half mayonnaise and half butter, or the oil may be calculated and mixed with the butter, depending on the child's taste and what makes food sense. In the case of hiding fat in ice cream, oil works nicely because it is liquid and has little flavor.

QUESTIONS AND ANSWERS

Q *How do you add extra ingredients to a meal plan when calculating by hand?*

A Take the tuna salad as an example. Suppose Jeremy wants to sprinkle baking chocolate shavings on his ice cream and bacon bits on the tuna salad. You would add a line for bacon and a line for baking chocolate in your hand or computer calculation. Then choose a small quantity, perhaps 5g of bacon and 2g of baking chocolate, and fill in the values for protein, fat, and carbohydrate of each. The quantities of other ingredients would then have to be juggled downward until all the columns add up to the proper totals. Bacon, which contains protein and fat, will take away from the meal's tuna and mayonnaise allotment. Baking chocolate, which is primarily fat and carbohydrate with a little protein, will take away from the amount of tomatoes in the meal. Because the overall carbohydrate allotment is very small, and the nutritive value of chocolate is less than that of vegetables, no more than 2g of chocolate should be used in a meal on the 4:1 ratio. With the accompanying computer program, an additional ingredient may simply be filled in on a blank line, and the other ingredients adjusted until the actual totals match the correctly prescribed ones.

Q *When is it necessary to make calorie adjustments?*

A Weight should be monitored on a weekly basis, and height on a monthly basis. Infants should be weighed and measured accurately at the pediatrician's office about every 2 weeks. At least during the fine-tuning period, the ketoteam should be informed monthly of a child's height and weight changes and any other relevant information. Once a child is started on the diet, changes in the diet order are usually made in response to her own performance—weight loss or gain, growth in height, seizure control, and other variables. We evaluate in this manner and may make adjustments based on these factors throughout her time on the diet.

Q *How often should a child eat on the ketogenic diet?*

A The number of meals and snacks included in a child's diet should approximate her pre-diet eating habits when possible, the family's schedule, and always take into account her nutritional needs. Infants will need to be given about six bottle feedings a day. Toddlers will probably need three meals and one or two snacks. Older children might need three meals and only one snack. Some children gain better overnight and achieve early morning seizure control by having a bedtime snack. Snacks are sometimes used to test how many extra calories a child who is losing weight needs and whether the extra calories cause any seizure activity problems.

SARAH WAS DOING WELL ON THE DIET, *eating three meals and one afternoon snack. Her seizures were virtually gone during the day, but she was still having seizures early every morning. At her follow-up check-up, the dietitian learned that Sarah was eating dinner at about 5:30P.M., going to bed around 7:30, and waking up at 7:00 for breakfast. It seemed that, in the 13.5 hours between dinner and breakfast, Sarah was running out of fats to make ketones! The dietitian offered the family the choice of having Sarah eating dinner later, or of having an evening snack. They decided on the snack. Once Sarah started eating her snack at bedtime, the early morning seizures disappeared.*

Q *Is it necessary to use half of the carbohydrate allotment as cream?*

A Using up to half of the carbohydrate allotment as cream is a guideline, not a hard and fast rule. Cream is an easy means to fit a lot of fat into the diet in a way that most children enjoy. If less cream is used, the child will have to eat more mayonnaise, butter, or oil. Some children like to eat fat, some don't. Some children love cream, some don't. As long as the diet makes food sense, there is no need to use half of the carbohydrate allotment as cream.

A DIET ORDER TEST

Lily is 24 months old and weighs 12 kilos. She is 86.5cm. tall. Both her height and weight are at the 50th percentile. She is going to start on a 4:1 ketogenic diet. What will her diet order read?

1.   At age two years, Lily's calorie per kilogram requirement will be approximately 75 calories per kilogram. (As indicated previously, calorie requirements vary with the metabolism and activity level of the child and must be individually assessed.) Her ideal weight is the same as her actual weight, 12 kilograms. So, Lily's total calorie

allotment is 75x12=900 calories per day.

2. Lily's dietary units will consist of 40 calories each, the standard for a 4:1 diet.

3. Lily's dietary units are determined by dividing her total calorie allotment by the calories in each dietary unit. So, she will have 900/40=22.5 dietary units per day.

4. Lily's daily fat allowance is determined by multiplying her dietary units (22.5) by the fat component in her ratio (4 in a 4:1 ratio). She will thus be allowed 22.5x4=90g fat per day.

5. Lily's protein+carbohydrate allotment is 22.5g per day, determined by multiplying her dietary units (22.5) by the 1 in her 4:1 ratio. As a young, growing child she may need 1.1 to 1.5g of protein/kg. Her weight is 12kg, so allowing 1.2g of protein per kilogram per day makes her protein allotment 14.4g per day.

6. Lily's daily carbohydrate allotment is determined by subtracting her protein allotment (14.4 g) from the total protein 1 carbohydrate allowance (22.5 g):22.5–14.4=8.1g carbohydrate per day.

Lily's complete diet order will read:

	PER DAY	PER MEAL
Protein	14.4g	4.8g
Fat	90.0g	30.0g
Carbohydrate	8.1g	2.7g
Calories	900	300

Note: As mentioned previously, most 2-year-olds eat one or twosnacks in addition to their three meals a day. This example has beensimplified for teaching purposes.

A MEAL TEST

For dinner, Lily would like to eat grilled chicken with fruit salad and a vanilla popsicle. How would you calculate this meal?

1. Start from the per-meal diet order. Lily is allowed a total of 2.7g carbohydrate per meal. To use half of this allotment as 36 percent cream, her popsicle should

contain 45g cream, which will provide 1.35g carbohydrate.

2. To provide her remaining 1.35g carbohydrate, she can have 13g of 10 percent fruit.

3. The 10 percent fruit and 36 percent cream contain a total of 1.03g protein. Lily's total protein allotment for the meal is 4.8g, so she can eat as much grilled chicken as will provide 4.8−1.03=3.77g protein. This works out to 12g chicken.

4. Lily is allowed 30g of fat in each meal. The chicken and cream contain a total of 16.5g fat. Lily should eat 17g of butter or mayonnaise to provide the additional 13.5g fat allotment.

CHICKEN CUTLET WITH FRUIT SALAD

	Weight	Protein	Fat	Carbo-hydrate	Calories
36% Cream	45g	0.9g	16.2g	1.4g	155
Chicken Breast	12g	3.7g	0.3g	—	18
10% Fruit Ex-change	13g	0. 1g	—	1.3g	6

Butter	17g	0.1g	13.8g	—	125
Actual Total		4.8g	30.3g	2.7g	304
Should Be		4.8g	30.0g	2.7g	300

Note: The chicken can be pounded very thin to make it look bigger on the plate. The fruit salad will be pretty if composed of small chunks of water-packed canned peaches and fresh strawberries. Lily thinks it is fun to pick up the chunks with a toothpick. The cream can be diluted with some allotted water, sweetened with saccharin, flavored with four or five drops of vanilla, and frozen in a popsicle mold in advance of the meal. Lily loves butter; she will eat it straight or it can be spread over her chicken. A small leaf of lettuce can be added to the meal for extra crunch.

CHAPTER THIRTEEN

LIQUID FORMULAS AND TUBE FEEDINGS

The ketogenic diet can be modified for all children, whether bottle-fed infants, small children making the transition from bottle to soft food, or children with special feeding problems. The ketogenic diet can be formulated in any texture—liquid, soft, solid, or a combination—and can be easily used even by children who need to be fed by nasogastric or gastrostomy tube. Two recent studies stress how easy, well-tolerated, and beneficial it can be to use the ketogenic diet as a formula-only treatment.

As discussed previously, seizures themselves, or the side effects of anticonvulsant medications, may affect a child's ability to eat properly. If the seizures are controlled or medications can be reduced using the ketogenic diet, the child may become able to come off soft or liquid diets after a time.

CALCULATING BOTH SOFT AND LIQUID DIETS

The process of calculating the diet, of establishing calorie levels and the grams of fat, protein, and carbohydrate permitted on the ketogenic diet, is the same regardless of the consistency of the food. The first steps in devising meal plans are the same as those used in calculating a traditional ketogenic diet: Follow the calculation process described in Chapter 12.

Remember, inactive children may need fewer calories per kilogram than average children. As always, monitor a child's weight closely for the first few months on the diet to make sure calories have been set at appropriate levels. This is of special importance in small infants.

Example

Emily was a 13-month-old girl admitted for the ketogenic diet in an attempt to achieve better control of her intractable seizures, which had continued despite heavy medication. She had been fed by gastrostomy tube since she was 8 months old. It was determined that she needed to lose weight; she was started on a 3:1 ratio at 70/kg and protein at 1.6/kg of desirable body weight.

Emily's age	13 months
Height	29.7" (76cm), 50th percentile for age
Actual weight	25 lb (11.4kg), 95th percentile for age
Ideal weight	21.5lb (9.8kg), 50th percentile for age
Calories/kg	70
Protein requirement	1.6g perkg of desirable body weight (Higher than used in older children
Ketogenic ratio	3:1

Using the above numbers in the formula described in Chapter 8, calculate the diet order via the following steps: (Note: Numbers are rounded to 0.1g.)

1. Calories: 70 (kcal/kg)x9.8 (kg ideal weight)=686 calories per day

2. Dietary unit: 686 (kcal)/31(kcal/dietary unit)=22.1 units per day
3. Fat allowance: 3 (as in 3:1)x22.1 (dietary units)=66.3g fat
4. Protein: 1.6 (grams perkg ideal weight)x9.8=15.7g protein
5. Carbohydrate: 22.1 (protein 1 carbohydrate)-15.7 (protein)=6.4g carbohydrate

Emily's daily diet order, which will be divided into the number of meals or bottles she regularly gets in a 24-hour period, will read:

	Daily
Protein	15.7g
Fat	66.3g
Carbohydrate	6.4g
Calories	686

PREPARING SOFT DIETS

Preparing the ketogenic diet in the form of soft, ground, or strained foods is really a question of texture rather than of theory, because the basic technique for formulating a soft-diet meal plan for tube feedings is the same as for solid foods. Commercial baby foods, like all commercially processed foods, should be checked to ensure that no added sugars are present.

For some children, the seizure reduction that comes with the ketogenic diet leads to changes in eating habits. For example, when Gabrielle first started the ketogenic diet, she was unable to swallow liquids without aspirating. She was on high doses of phenobarbital and was having more than a hundred seizures a day. She could eat soft foods, but liquids had to be given through a gastrostomy tube.

Within 4 months of diet initiation, Gabrielle became almost seizurefree (except when she was sick). She was tapered off her phenobarbital and, as she came off the medication, grew more alert. A swallow study showed that she could now be fed by mouth and discontinue the gastrostomy tube.

PREPARING LIQUID OR TUBE FEEDINGS

The ketogenic diet in liquid form is used primarily for infants and for children who are fed by gastrostomy tube. The process of calculating allotted protein, carbohydrate, and fat is the same for liquid diets as for diets of other consistencies.

Liquid ketogenic diets are most often composed of three ingredients:

- Ross Carbohydrate-free (RCF) concentrate

    —Soy-based protein, avoids symptoms of cow's milk sensitivities

    —Available through Ross in a concentrated liquid: 13 fluid ounce cans; 12 per case; No.108

- Microlipid (Mead Johnson)

    A safflower-oil emulsion that mixes easily in solution; made by Mead Johnson

    —Rich source of polyunsaturated fat and high in linoleic acid

    —Available in 90mL bottles; 24 per case; product code 8884-300400

- Polycose powder (glucose polymers)

    —Source of calories derived solely from carbohydrate

    —Available through Ross in powder form (350g cans); 6 per case; No.746.

Carbohydrate-free multivitamins and minerals, calcium supplements, and sterile water are added to complete the mixture.

FOOD VALUES FOR LIQUID DIET CALCULATION

	Quantity	Protein	Fat	Carbohy-drate
RCF Con-centrate	100cc	4.0g	7.2g	—
Microlipid	100cc	—	50.0g	—
Canola Oil	100g	—	97.1g	—
Polycose Powder	100g	—	—	94.0g

Because it is emulsified, Microlipid mixes more easily with the other ingredients than oil and is easier to digest. But Microlipid is also more expensive than corn oil or canola oil. Vegetable oil may be used for larger (older) children or when expense is a factor. MCT oil may also be added to a formula if the dietitian thinks it is needed, for example to loosen stools or boost ketosis.

SETTING UP A LIQUID MEAL PLAN

1. Calculate the amount of RCF needed to satisfy the child's protein requirement by cross-multiplying.

   Emily's desirable weight is 9.8 kilograms. Her protein requirement is 1.6g per kilogram of desirable body weight, or 1.6x9.8=15.7g per day. 100g of RCF formula contains 4.0g of protein. Use the following formula:

   $$\frac{100}{4.0} = \frac{X}{15.7} = \frac{100 \times 15.7}{4.0} = 393 \text{ cc}$$

   Emily will need 393cc RCF concentrate to meet her 15.7g protein requirement.

2. Calculate the fat in RCF by cross-multiplying, and calculate enough Microlipid to make up the difference.

   100g RCF contains 7.2g fat. Emily's 393cc of RCF contains:

   $$\frac{100}{7.2} = \frac{393}{X} = \frac{393 \times 7.2}{100} \text{ or } 28.3 \text{ g fat}$$

Subtract the 28.3g fat from the total 66.4g fat needed (66.4–28.3=38.1). Remaining fat is 38.1g.

3. To calculate the Microlipid needed to make up the remaining 37.4g fat in Emily's diet, cross-multiply.

$$\frac{100}{50} = \frac{X}{38.1} = \frac{100 \times 38.1}{50} = X, X = 76.2 \text{ cc Microlipid}$$

4. Calculate an amount of Polycose powder sufficient to meet Emily's carbohydrate requirement.

100g Polycose powder contains 94.0g carbohydrate. Emily needs 6.8g Polycose powder to provide her required 6.4g carbohydrate, determined by the following formula:

$$\frac{100}{94} = \frac{X}{6.4} = \frac{100 \times 6.4}{94} \text{ or 6.8 g}$$

5. The liquid allotment is set at 100mL per kilogram of desirable body weight, giving Emily 980mL liquid per day.

Emily's RCF and Microlipid total 469.2cc (393 RCF+76.2 Microlipid). Her water allotment will therefore be 980−469.2=510.8cc. This will be rounded to 511cc.

EMILY'S DAILY FORMULA

	Quantity	Protein	Fat	Carbohy-drate
RCF con-centrate	393cc	15.7g	28.3g	—
Microlipid	76.2cc	—	38.1g	—
Polycose powder	6.8g	—	—	6.4g
Sterile water	511cc	—	—	—
Total	987cc	15.7g	66.4g	6.4 g

Note: In practice, this meal would be rounded to the nearest gram for convenience in measuring.

PREPARATION OF KETOGENIC LIQUID FORMULA

1. Measure the RCF concentrate and Microlipid separately in a graduated cylinder.
2. Weigh the Polycose powder on a gram scale and blend with above ingredients.
3. Add sterile water, reserving 10 to 15cc per feeding to flush the tube. Shake or stir.

4. Divide into the number of equal feedings the child will receive in a 24-hour period and refrigerate, or refrigerate full amount and divide into individual portions at feeding time.

5. Bring to room temperature or warm slightly before feeding.

6. *Note:* Remember to supplement this formula with vitamins and minerals.

Liquid feedings may be given orally or through tubes. They may be given by continuous drip or as periodic feedings. The tubes may be flushed with 10 to 15cc of sterile or tap water, but no more than this because of the diet's fluid restrictions.

Some families reserve some of the water for between meal feedings. This is also acceptable, as long as the child receives the total amount of fluid.

Children on liquid feedings who do not have a swallowing difficulty, such as growing babies, may be "transitioned" to soft foods by gradually substituting the equivalent soft foods for a portion of their bottle feedings. The liquid ketogenic formula is relatively expensive. However, since the liquid ketogenic diet is considered a therapy rather than a food, WIC programs and many insurance companies will cover its cost. The following sample letter may be of help in communicating the reasons for the diet:

WIC Program

Case Review Services

Re: Ketogenic Diet Therapy

For: _____

DOB: _____

Attention Case Manager:

_____ is a _____-month old boy/girl with a diagnosis of _____ and an intractable seizure disorder. His seizures were occurring _____ times each day despite attempts at seizure control with _____ (name anticonvulsants here).

The ketogenic diet is a high-fat, adequate-protein, low-carbohydrate formula that is individually calculated and prescribed to produce adequate ketosis to suppress the child's seizures. The formula, which is fed by (bottle/gastrostomy tube) is comprised of Ross carbohydrate-free formula, Polycose powder, and Microlipid made by the MeadJohnson Company. The formula must be supplemented with multivitamins and minerals in order to be nutritionally complete.

We are requesting that, since these components constitute an antiepileptic therapy rather than just a nutritional formula, they be covered under your policies.

Thank you for helping _____ to develop as free of seizures and medications as possible.

Sincerely,

KETOCAL

Over the past decade, SHS International (Liverpool, UK) has created a pre-prepared, nutritionally complete, ketogenic formula called Keto-Cal™. It is approved for children over 1 year of age but, in many ketogenic diet centers, it is used for infants as well. This vanilla tasting, powdered formula is designed to create a 4:1 ketogenic diet in liquid form. While a 3:1 ratio KetoCal is currently not available in the United States, the current 4:1 ratio can be converted readily to a 3:1. Contact SHS North America (Rockville, MD: 1-800-365-7354; Canada: 877-636-2283) for further details.

Calories must be calculated for each child. KetoCal is composed of 90 percent fat, 8.4 percent protein, and 1.6 percent carbohydrates by calories. The formula can be given orally or via gastrostomy tube, and tastes better if chilled. We have used it for some of our patients on the Atkins diet as a meal replacement and as a method to give a slight boost to ketones (see Chapter 15). Once the can has been opened, it should be used or discarded after 1 month.

The following instructions are provided courtesy of SHS International and are available on their website: htt p://www.shsna.com/pages/ketocal.htm:

INSTRUCTIONS:

Measure the required amount of warm water into a container that seals with a screw top lid. To completely dissolve the powder, the water must be at a temperature of 113 to 122°F.

Add the prescribed amount of KetoCal to the water.

Cover and shake until the powder has dissolved.

Once prepared, the formula should be stored in a refrigerator and kept no longer than 24 hours. KetoCal can be kept at room temperature for a maximum of 4 hours.

Shake or stir immediately before serving. For oral feeding, KetoCal is best served chilled.

To obtain the recommended dilution of 4mL of water to 1g of powder, mix the following amounts of water and powder:

WATER	POWDER	FINAL VOLUME	KCAL/ML
80mL	20g	100mL	1.44
400mL	100g	500mL	1.44
800mL	200g	1,000mL	1.44

A gram scale is necessary for proper preparation of formula.

To order, contact SHS at 1-800-365-7354 or nutritionservices @shsna.com.

The mailing address for SHS is:
HS North America
P.O. Box 117
Gaithersburg, MD 20884

SECTION IV
MODIFIED KETOGENIC DIETS

CHAPTER FOURTEEN

THE MCT DIET

WE HAVE ALREADY BEEN ON THE KETOGENIC DIET ONCE. We used that MCT oil stuff, and it was awful. Our daughter had terrible diarrhea and the seizures didn't improve, so we stopped after 2 weeks. Why would you suggest that we consider trying it again?

—TP

In the mid-20th century, when the diet was falling into disuse because of new anticonvulsants and a feeling that the diet was unpalatable, Dr. Peter Huttenlocher of the University of Chicago tried to invent a new and improved form of ketogenic diet. He believed that the ketogenic diet was an effective form of therapy and that more families would try—and benefit from—a ketogenic diet if it were formulated with foods more closely approximating a normal diet.

Dr. Huttenlocher's team called their formulation the MCT diet, for "medium-chain triglycerides." They replaced the long-chain triglycerides of the fats in the classic ketogenic diet—fats found in butter, mayonnaise, olive oil, and most other dietary fats—with medium-chain triglycerides, which have shorter molecular chain lengths.

Medium-chain triglycerides (MCT) are found as an odorless, colorless, tasteless oil. MCTs have to be calculated into the diet just like any other fat, but medium-chain triglycerides are more ketogenic than longchain triglycerides. Therefore, an MCT diet with calories at 100 percent of RDA levels, and with more carbohydrates and protein, will produce the same urinary ketosis as a classic ketogenic diet with calories at 75 percent of RDA levels.

MCT oil can thus be said to be "more ketogenic" than other dietary fats. Because the diet is more ketogenic, a child on the MCT diet can eat a wider variety of other, anti-ketogenic foods, such as larger portions of fruit and vegetables and even a small amount of bread and other starches. Fluids are not restricted on this diet. Dr. Huttenlocher and his colleagues hoped that a more palatable diet, that allowed a wider variety of foods, would foster greater compliance from children and families and make it easier for a child to have a more normal life while maintaining ketosis.

The MCT diet, like the classic ketogenic diet, is initiated after a brief fast and usually shows results within several days of its inception. Children must stick with it just as rigidly as with the classic ketogenic diet. If the MCT diet works, children similarly stay on it for about 2 years.

WHY THEN USE THE STANDARD KETOGENIC DIET?

A comparison of the classic ketogenic diet with the MCT diet and a modified ketogenic diet (Table 3-2) found all three to be equally effective in achieving seizure control. Compliance and palatability, however, were found to be better with the classic ketogenic diet.

Although the MCT diet has been reported to be equally effective as the classic ketogenic diet, this has not been our experience at Johns Hopkins. We have found that the MCT diet is usually too high in calories (thus providing inferior seizure control) and is not more palatable than the classic diet. In fact, our experience indicates that ingestion of the MCT oil is often accompanied by abdominal cramps, severe and persistent diarrhea, or nausea and vomiting. If children cannot hold it down, it cannot be effective. We often supplement the "classic" ketogenic diet with small amounts of MCT oil, both because it can increase ketosis and because it may decrease the constipation that often accompanies the ketogenic diet.

Some parents or physicians may want to try the MCT diet for children, perhaps with the thought of providing a higher volume of food. If the child does not have trouble with the oil, and if the seizures are completely controlled, some families appreciate the additional anti-ketogenic calories that the MCT diet affords. If the MCT diet does not work, or if it is not tolerated, we recommend trying the classic ketogenic diet.

Many parents tell us that their child has already been on the ketogenic diet without success. On further questioning, this prior diet often turns out to have been the MCT diet. We have found some children who continued to have seizures despite tolerating the MCT diet, but who subsequently responded well to the classic ketogenic diet. We have also seen many children and families who could not tolerate the MCT diet but who did well on the classic ketogenic diet. In other words, we at Hopkins have found that a little imagination applied to the classic ketogenic diet is more effective and more palatable than is the MCT formulation.

CHAPTER FIFTEEN

USING THE ATKINS DIET FOR EPILEPSY

During the mid 1990s, as the ketogenic diet was being rediscovered, Dr. Robert C. Atkins wrote an editorial pointing out similarities between the ketogenic diet and his Atkins diet. Both are high in fats and low in carbohydrates, and both produce ketosis. There are, however, important differences:

- The primary goal of the Atkins diet is weight loss, whereas the goal of the ketogenic diet is seizure control.
- The Atkins diet does not have restricted calories or fluids, and does not require a fast or a hospital admission to implement.

If the Atkins diet produces ketosis but is easier for children to tolerate and families to implement, we wondered if it could be used, like the ketogenic diet, in the treatment of epilepsy.

Kate, a 7-year-old-girl, provided a chance to test this theory. Kate was 1 month away from her scheduled admission for initiation of the ketogenic diet. Her seizures were occurring 70 to 80 times per day, and she had failed eight anticonvulsants. In preparation for her ketogenic diet initiation, we suggested a gradual reduction of high-carbohydrate foods, such as bread, pizza, cake, and breakfast cereal, to get her accustomed to the foods that would be given on the diet. Kate's mother asked for more information about reducing carbohydrates, so we suggested that she buy the Atkins diet book, *Dr. Atkins' New Diet Revolution,* and read about the Atkins diet's induction phase. Kate's mother bought the book on a Friday. By Monday, Kate's seizures had totally stopped.

When we saw Kate in clinic, her urine ketones were large, just as if she had been on the ketogenic diet. Our dietitian calculated that Kate was receiving about 10g per day of carbohydrates, similar to what children her size would be permitted on the ketogenic diet. After 1 month of seizure-freedom, we cancelled her admission. Although Kate continued to have occasional seizures, mostly with illnesses, she was able to cut her medications in half and decrease her seizures by more than 90 percent on the Atkins diet.

Since our experience with Kate, we at Johns Hopkins have started a number of children on a modified Atkins diet, with the goal of producing ketosis in a less restrictive manner that is easier on children and their families than is the ketogenic diet. Not only does the Atkins diet not restrict protein, calories, or fluids, pre-made Atkins diet products are available in many grocery stores and restaurants. The Atkins diet also allows a child to choose items off a menu at a school cafeteria or restaurant, which is nearly impossible on the ketogenic diet.

Of the first six children we studied on the Atkins-like diet, three had a greater than 90 percent reduction in seizures, and four stayed on the diet more than 3 months. In a recently completed study of 20 children with difficult-to-control seizures, 14, or 65 percent, had a greater than 50 percent reduction in seizures. Half of those (35 percent of the twenty children) had a greater than 90 percent reduction in seizures. Many were on fewer medications at the end of the study and decided to stay on past the 6-month study period. These results appeared to be similar to the results we achieved on the ketogenic diet.

Our dietitian estimates that the Atkins diet is approximating a 1.5 to 2:1 fat to carbohydrate ratio, compared with a 4:1 or 3:1 ratio in the classic ketogenic diet. The children we studied who used the Atkins diet to control seizures did *not* lose weight on the Atkins diet; their body mass index remained stable. Seizure control seemed to remain even when urinary ketosis fluctuated. No child got kidney stones. About 1 in 5 children using the Atkins diet for seizure control experienced constipation, and 1 in 3 had hunger issues even without calorie restriction. Most of the children who went up from 10 to 20g of carbohydrates per day did fine. In a current study here at Johns

Hopkins, we're trying to find out which starting carbohydrate amount is best.

Although the potential ease of the Atkins diet relative to the ketogenic diet is appealing, it is only beginning to be studied. Key questions remain as to whether it is as effective as the ketogenic diet, and whether it is in fact easier to use for seizure control than the ketogenic diet.

Most families using the Atkins diet for epilepsy still need lots of help from our staff, as well as turning to each other for support, recipes, and advice. It's best to do some reading, too. Good books include the one you are reading now, *Dr. Atkins New Diet Revolution,* and *The 2005 Doctor's Pocket Calorie, Fat, & Carb Counter,* along with any recipe book of low-carbohydrate recipes. The Internet is another good source (e.g., www.atkins.com and www.atkinsforseizures.com).

TABLE15-1: Differences Between the Ketogenic and a Modified Atkins Diet

	Ketogenic Diet	Modified Atkins
Calories (% recommended daily allowance)	Restricted (75%)	Unrestricted

Fluids	Restricted (80%)	Unrestricted
Fat	80%	60%
Protein	15%	30%
Carbohydrates	5%	10%
Multiple studies over many years proving benefits	Yes	No

HOW TO USE A MODIFIED ATKINS DIET FOR EPILEPSY

Based on the children (and a few adults) whose epilepsy we have treated using the Atkins diet, we believe that, like the original ketogenic diet, it should be started, monitored, and stopped under medical or dietetic supervision.

Starting the diet: the first month

We strongly suggest that, before they begin, families who wish to start using the Atkins diet for control of seizures discuss their plans with their physician or neurologist, and obtain baseline information on height and weight, blood work including liver and kidney functions and lipids, and urine testing for calcium and creatinine. To get an accurate picture of the diet's effectiveness, medications should not be changed for 2 to 3 weeks before starting the diet. A desired weight may be set if weight loss or weight gain is an issue.

During the first several days, as with ketogenic diet initiation, some children quickly become too ketotic and display symptoms of sleepiness, dehydration, or vomiting. Some may even require hospital admission for intravenous fluids (in many cases a little bit of orange juice can help the ketones get back in balance). Addressing these problems is one reason for maintaining close contact with a physician as the Atkins diet is started.

When starting the Atkins diet for epilepsy:

- We suggest starting carbohydrates at 10g per day for children and 15g per day for adolescents. However, we are still learning the best starting point for ketosis and tolerability.

- Children should take a sugar-free multivitamin such as Unicap M™, and a daily calcium supplement such as Calci-Mix.
- Urinary ketones should be tested two or three times per week (or whenever seizures are increasing for no apparent reason) using Bayer Ketostix™.

Typical 2 Days of Food for a Child on a Carbohydrate 10g/day Modified Atkins Diet

Day 1
Breakfast
Scrambled eggs
Bacon (2 strips)
36% heavy whipping cream diluted with water to make milk
Lunch
Bologna/ham, lettuce, Dijon mayonnaise "roll-ups"
Raspberries (1/2 cup)
Cucumber slices (1/2 cup)
Flavored, calorie-free, sparkling water
Snack
Just the cheese™ (crunchy) snacks

Dinner

Hot dog

Spaghetti squash with butter and salt (1/4 cup)

Day 2

Breakfast

Sausage links

Low carbohydrate yogurt

Water

Lunch

Cheeseburger (no bun)

Cole slaw

Pickle

Heavy whipping cream, water, and unsweetened cocoa powder

Snack

5 macadamia nuts

Mozzarella cheese stick

Dinner

Sliced chicken, coated in egg and CarbSense™ baking mix, then fried in olive oil Steamed, mashed cauliflower with salt, butter, and pepper (mashed "potatoes") 1/2 cup of strawberries topped with heavy whipping cream

- Weight should be checked every week, and the physician or dietitian should be consulted if significant weight loss or gain occurs.

For the first month, store-bought, low-carbohydrate products should be avoided and medications left unchanged.

MAINTAINING THE ATKINS DIET FOR EPILEPSY: HELPFUL HINTS

After the first month, maintenance on the Atkins diet for epilepsy is similar to that for the ketogenic diet. If seizure control is less than desirable, fat sources, such as mayonnaise, butter, heavy cream, or oil, including MCT oil, can be used. If a child is too ketotic (sleepy or lacking energy), carbohydrates can be increased slightly. The following are some additional ways of adjusting the diet if additional seizure control is needed:

- **Avoid sugar alcohols.** Loss of ketosis and increased seizures can occur after eating a low-carbohydrate candy bar or shake. Read labels carefully to avoid any products with excessive sugar alcohols (e.g. maltitol, xylitol). Only a maximum of one new low-carb product should be eaten per day. Do not serve packaged food for which no label information on carbohydrates is provided and which is not in your carbohydrate counter book.

- **Give the full amount of carbohydrates.** The 10 to 15g of carbohydrate allowed on the diet should not be diminished, and it should come primarily in the form of fruits and vegetables, which provide important nutrients and fiber content to avoid constipation.
- **Don't overdo artificial sweeteners in powder form.** Most powdered sweeteners are mixed with corn starch to make them powders. Enough packets mixed to make a punch drink can provide too many carbohydrates and throw off ketosis.
- **Space food throughout the day.** Spacing meals and snacks throughout the day can be helpful for maintaining ketosis and avoiding hunger.

- **Supplement fat sources if necessary.** Fats are an important part of any ketogenic diet for epilepsy. Butter, mayonnaise, oil, and cream are an important part of the Atkins diet and should be used liberally. If a boost in ketosis is still needed, additives may be used. MCT oil, which is dense with fats, can be given as a supplement with meals to boost ketones. Also, SHS KetoCal™ is a powder with a 4:1 ratio that can be mixed with water to create a vanilla shake and boost ketones.

- **Subtract "absorbed" carbohydrates.** To calculate "absorbed" carbohydrates, subtract fiber from total carbohydrates on the label. Fiber is not absorbed and can be ignored from a carbohydrate point of view.

- **Patience, patience, patience.** Many of our children and adults did *not* see improvement until past 3 months on the Atkins diet. This happens with the ketogenic diet, too. Make only one change at a time, and give the diet at least 3 months. If you've come this far, give it a chance.

- **Make it a family affair.** Some of our most compliant children came from families in which the mother and father also cut carbohydrates. It's not necessary to be too restrictive, but getting cakes, cookies, breakfast cereal, and juices out of the house can help tremendously. In some cases, spouses of our adult patients lost weight and became some of our best supporters.

- **All-natural is not the same as ketogenic.** Many health food stores carry low carbohydrate products nowadays. They also carry foods that are organic, all-natural, vegetarian, and high-carbohydrate. Although some of these products might be acceptable on the Atkins diet, often they are not acceptable. Always read the labels.

- **Get help.** One of the biggest lessons from our studies was that, although the Atkins diet was easier to carry out than the ketogenic diet, it is still hard! Several of our families interacted via phone and e-mail and shared support, recipes, and good ideas. This has made a difference for many families, especially because the Atkins diet, by its very design, requires less hospital support. The website http://www.atkinsforseizures.com is very useful; it was created and is being run by one of our parents.

DISCONTINUING THE ATKINS DIET

Should the diet not appear to be helping, it can be stopped quite easily. We recommend a test of the diet's effectiveness before discontinuing it: Give a glass of liquid sweetened by sugar (such as juice or soda) and watch for a drop in ketones. If this leads to worsening of seizures, the Atkins diet may be more helpful than originally believed.

Once the decision has been made to stop the diet, increase carbohydrates slowly by 10g every 3 to 4 days, and follow ketones daily until they disappear. At that point, go back to a regular diet.

CONCLUSION

Although the benefits of the Atkins diet for treating difficult-to-control epilepsy are not yet well documented, we are impressed with the promise of the diet for epilepsy. It may be that only some, but not all children need the high ketogenic ratio and restricted calories and liquids provided by the ketogenic diet in order to achieve good seizure control. Perhaps some children will achieve good results using the Atkins diet, and others may get better results with the classical ketogenic diet. Some families may choose to try the Atkins approach first because of its relative ease of use and the fact that it does not involve a hospital admission. If seizure control is less than desirable, a family can always try the ketogenic diet later.

SECTION V
KETOGENIC COOKING

CHAPTER SIXTEEN

SAMPLE MEAL PLANS FOR THE KETOGENIC DIET

Although quantities are limited and smaller than a child is used to, the variety and appeal of food on the ketogenic diet is limited only by your creativity!

- Filet of beef with strawberry cream popsicle
- Eggs Benedict
- Cheese omelet with orange juice
- Shrimp scampi with pumpkin parfait
- Cheesecake

Nearly all the foods your child likes can be transformed into a ketogenic meal. The ketogenic diet can be such a gift—the meals need not be considered a punishment!

AS OFTEN AS POSSIBLE, *Michael has something that we are having. If I am making pork chops for us, I cook him one. If we are* *having tuna fish sandwiches, he has tuna fish with mayonnaise wrapped in a leaf of lettuce.*

—EH

Parents should not stray from the basic meal plans in the beginning, for the sake of simplicity and control while learning how to implement the diet and whether ketosis provides effective seizure control for their child. When the diet has been proven useful, and they are familiar with its preparation, parents can begin to get more creative with flavorings and new menu plans.

Herbs and spices, lemon juice, soy sauce, baking chocolate, catsup, and other flavorings all contain carbohydrates. The overall carbohydrate level in the diet is extremely low, so that catsup calculated into a meal plan may eliminate your child's fruit or vegetable allotment. Herbs and spices should be limited to a tiny pinch and high-carbohydrate flavorings, such as catsup or chocolate, should only be used occasionally if at all.

Pure vanilla flavoring, up to five drops a meal, has no countable food value and can be considered "free," which is to say not affecting the ketogenic balance of the meal. Other pure, carbohydrate-free extracts, such as almond, lemon, or chocolate, are similarly "free."

IT WAS IMPORTANT TO MY SON to feel as though he was getting a dessert. So I always kept a stock of homemade cream popsicles in the freezer, flavored with vanilla or chocolate (which was calculated into his meal plans) and a little bit of saccharin. He got one after every dinner. If he was supposed to have 80cc of cream and the Tupperware Popsicle molds only held 60cc, he drank the rest of the cream straight.

—CC

Think of the recipes included in this chapter in terms of entire meal plans, not as single food items. The ketogenic ratio of food in the diet must balance within a whole meal, so any food calculated into one part of the meal affects what can go into other parts.

The menus that follow are examples drawn from the experience of various parents and are for a "generic" child. Your own meal plans will take into account your child's calorie level, protein needs, ketogenic ratio, and individual preferences. When a child has been seizure-free for a year, and your physician allows the ketogenic ratio to be lowered to 3:1, larger portions of meat, fruit, and vegetables will be allowed to balance against less fat and cream, thus permitting greater variety and flexibility.

GO TO RESTAURANTS! Eat together as a family! Enjoy the benefits you get from the diet. Try not to segregate your child or feed her separately from the rest of the family. She will enjoy feeling included. Most kids appreciate the reduction of seizures and freedom from medication more than they covet the food they cannot eat!

—CC

TIPS

The following are tips from parents who have experienced the ketogenic diet:

- Kids don't mind eating the same thing over and over. Find several simple menus that you and your child can agree on, and stick with them. Six to eight menus is probably all you'll need. The multivitamin and calcium will take care of the rest!
- Use a salad plate so the amount of food seems larger.
- Fix a few meals in advance and keep them in the refrigerator in carefully labeled Tupperware containers (breakfast, lunch, etc.) in case you are not there at mealtimes, or for when your child goes to school or to a friend's house. You will build up a huge Tupperware collection.
- Processed meats are a poor source of protein and can affect a child's ability to maintain good ketosis. Minimize the use of packaged or processed foods.

- Use the speck of spices that are allowed (but remember they do contain carbohydrate). A small amount goes a long way toward making the food interesting.
- My son will drink the cream straight down, but I often mix it with sugar-free soda so that it will fill him up more.
- Steam vegetables to provide the best nutrition and keep water weight out of the food.
- Save a couple of favorite meals for extra special times. Use these meals less than once a week so that they remain special for times when you are having something your child loves but cannot have, or for times when nothing else sounds good.
- Chopped lettuce with mayonnaise can be a fairly large-looking element of a meal. It really helps fill up the plate, and it helps with bowel movements.
- Find places to hide the fat. Oil hides well in applesauce or ice cream. Butter disappears into peanut butter or cream cheese. Tuna, chicken, or egg salad eats up mayonnaise.

- Select dishes that are familiar and resemble your family's normal meals.
- Don't assume that a zero-calorie powdered drink is OK. Many contain carbohydrates such as maltodextrin. Always read labels carefully!
- Don't mix nasty-tasting medicine or supplements with food. Separate medicines from food as much as possible. Sometimes sprinkles of medicines can be mixed in as long as your child can't taste it.
- Do not buy diet foods—use real mayonnaise, butter, eggs, and so on. Diet foods tend to have high water content and extra carbohydrates.
- Counter the small quantity of food with creative shapes and arrangements: slice meat thinly and fan it out. Pound chicken paper-thin. Cut carrots into carrot chips, cucumbers into shoestring sticks.

BASIC TECHNIQUES

The recipes in this chapter do not show quantities, because these must be calculated for each individual child. Each recipe is for a whole meal, considered as a unit, because foods in one part of the meal affect what can be included in another part while maintaining the prescribed ketogenic ratio. As a rule, ingredients such as catsup, lemon juice, vinegar, herbs and spices, soy sauce, and baking chocolate are used in very small quantities (such as 2 g, or about 1/8 teaspoon).

Meats should be lean with fat removed. Fish and poultry should be skinless and boneless. This is to ensure that the child's protein allotment is as close to pure or solid protein as possible.

Cooked foods should be trimmed and weighed on theg scale after cooking, except in the case of food that is heated only slightly or will not change volume during cooking (such as cheese for melting or eggs). Previously cooked foods do not have to be weighed again after reheating.

The exchange list in Table 16-1 shows whether a specific vegetable should be weighed raw or cooked. "What the eye sees, the mind remembers," the old adage goes. But food amounts should not be "guesstimated." You may get used to judging how much 25g of chicken or 15g of applesauce is, but you should always check with a scale for accuracy. The quantity of each ingredient in these menus varies from child to child, so we have not given exact amounts here. Quantities can be calculated either by hand or by using a computer program in consultation with a doctor or dietitian.

EXCHANGE LISTS

In the hand-calculated ketogenic diet, fruits and vegetables with similar carbohydrate contents have been grouped into lists of items that may be substituted for one another interchangeably (Table 16-1).

Exchange Lists

FRUIT OR JUICE: FRESH OR CANNED WITHOUT SUGAR			
10% (Use amount prescribed)		15% (Use 2/3 amount prescribed)	
Applesauce, Mott's	Papaya	Apple	Kiwi
Cantaloupe	Peach	Apricot	Mango
Grapefruit	Strawberries	Blackberries	Nectarine
Grapes, purple	Tangerine	Blueberries	Pear
Honeydew melon	Watermelon	Figs	Pineapple
Orange	Grapes, green	Raspberries	

VEGETABLES: FRESH, CANNED, OR FROZEN
Measure Raw (R) or Cooked (C) as Specified

Group A (Use twice amount prescribed)		Group B (Use amount prescribed)	
Asparagus/C	Radish/R	Beets/C	Kohlrabi/C
Beet greens/C	Rhubarb/R	Broccoli/C	Mushroom/R
Cabbage/C	Sauerkraut/C	Brussels sprouts/C	Mustard greens/C
Celery/C or R	Summer squash/C	Cabbage/R	Okra/C
Chicory/R	Swiss chard/C	Carrots/R or C	Onion/R or C
Cucumbers/R	Tomato/R	Cauliflower/C	Rutabaga/C
Eggplant/C	Tomato juice	Collards/C	Spinach/C
Endive/R	Turnips/C	Dandelion greens/C	Tomato/C
Green pepper/R or C	Turnip greens/C	Green beans/C	Winter squash/C
Poke/C	Watercress/R	Kale/C	

FAT
Unsaturated fats are recommended

Butter	Canola oil	Flaxseed oil	Margarine
Corn oil	Peanut oil	Mayonnaise	Olive oil

When a menu calls for 21g of 10 percent fruit, you may choose cantaloupe, orange, strawberry, peach, or any other item from the 10 percent fruit list. Or you may choose to use 14g (two-thirds the amount prescribed) of a 15 percent fruit, such as blueberries, pear, or pineapple. Similarly, if a menu calls for 18g of a Group B vegetable, you may choose any item or combination of items from the Group B list, including broccoli, mushrooms, or green beans. Or you may choose to use twice that amount, 36g, of any Group A vegetable or combination of Group A vegetables, including asparagus, celery, and summer squash.

All the other ingredients in the diet, including meats, fats, and cheeses, should be specified individually in each menu.

Exchange lists allow greater flexibility in using fruits and vegetables. The diet works well with this method, in spite of minor variations in the makeup of each vegetable and fruit. If a child is eating exclusively highcarbohydrate fruits and vegetables, such as grapes and carrots, menus should be calculated specifically for these items.

When hand calculation was the norm, meats, fats, and cheeses were also used in generic exchange list form. In spite of significant variations in the content of items on each exchange list, this worked well for some children who could tolerate the resulting fluctuation in diet content. In an effort to provide optimal ketosis for the greatest number of children, and with the more precise computer menu planning now the norm, only fruit and vegetables are now used in generic exchange list form.

"FREE"WAYS TO DRESS UP YOUR CREAM

Ice cream ball	• Dust with a speck of cinnamon or nutmeg
	• Flavor with sweetener and vanilla or calculated baking chocolate
	• Whip in canola oil after 1 hour of freezing
	• Flavor with sweetener and vanilla or calculated baking chocolate
Whipped parfait	• Layer with calculated berries
	• Sprinkle with a chopped nut
	• Flavor with sweetener and vanilla, lemon, maple, almond, or
	• Serve on top of calculated sugar-free Jell-O
Cream soda	• Pour cream into fruit-flavored sugar-free soda

Note: The following meal plans must be prepared using the calculatedfood amount specified for an individual child.

DON'T FORGET SUPPLEMENTS. The ketogenic diet must be supplemented with a sugarless multi-vitamin and mineral, and a calcium supplement every day.

SCRAMBLED EGG BREAKFAST

Egg

Butter

Cream

Orange juice

Options (The following must be calculated into the meal plan if desired)

Crisp bacon, ham, or sausage

Grated cheese in omelettes

Vegetables, fresh fruit, or applesauce instead of juice

Baking chocolate for cocoa

Beat equal amounts of yolk and white. Cook eggs in a microwave or nonstick pan, which may be sprayed with nonstick vegetable oil. Transfer to scale and weigh, trimming if necessary. Transfer to plate and add any additional butter. For omelettes, egg should be cooked flat and thin, then put back in pan, filled with calculated cheese or vegetable/butter mixture, heated slightly, and scraped thoroughly onto a plate with a small rubber spatula. Garnish plate with calculated crisp bacon and/or grated cheese sprinkles. Dilute cream with water or ice to make it more like milk, or make hot chocolate by melting baking chocolate shavings in cream with sweetener. Your child must consume all the butter on the plate. Drink orange juice or eat fruit last for dessert. If you choose to include bacon or cheese, less egg will be allowed in the meal plan, because the protein allotment will be shared.

KETO PANCAKES

Egg
Butter
Sugar-free sweetener Cottage cheese
Cream
Fresh fruit slices

Beat egg white until stiff. Fold in yolk, cottage cheese, and sweetener. Spray nonstick pan with cooking spray. Pour mixture into pan to form a round disk about 3/4-inch thick. Cook thoroughly on first side before turning (or the pancake will fall apart). Top with "syrup" made of melted butter mixed with a few drops of sweetener and carbohydrate-free pure maple flavoring. Serve with fruit slices on the side.

WESTERN OMELETTE

Egg
Mayonnaise
Green pepper
Dill, basil, salt, pepper Cream
Tomato
Onion

Scramble egg and weigh. Add a little of allotted cream and scramble again. Pour into heated pan coated with vegetable cooking spray. Chop vegetables. Sprinkle with pinch of spices. Mix with mayonnaise. Spread vegetable/mayonnaise mixture on egg. Then flip top over to make omelet and cook a few more minutes until done. This omelet may also be made in a sandwich machine by pouring half of the egg on the grid, spreading the vegetable mixture on top, then adding the other half of the egg and closing the machine until done.

EASY APPLE-SAUSAGE BAKE

Unsweetened applesauce
Butter
Sweetener, vanilla
Bob Evans sausage link
Cream
Speck of cinnamon

Broil sausage link under medium flame until brown, boil until done, or sauté in frying pan. Drain on paper towel. Weigh and trim. Meanwhile, place applesauce in small ovenproof container. Mix in brown sugar substi-tute or sweetener, top with butter, and place under broiler. Whip cream until it thickens, add a few drops of vanilla and sweetener, and continue beating until stiff. When applesauce is warm and butter is melted, top with whipped cream and dust with cinnamon. Serve with sausage.

APPLESAUCE is a great place to hide fat. As much as equal parts fat to applesauce will blend in and taste good. Add a 1/4-grain of saccharin dissolved in warm water or a dash of liquid sweetener to unsweetened applesauce and dust with a speck of cinnamon before serving. May be served warm or at room temperature.

PEANUT BUTTER MUFFINS

4:1, 120 calories per three muffins
9g egg
8g butter
4g Skippy peanut butter
Whip whites until stiff, add yolk, measure 9g. Melt butter and peanut butter in microwave and add to egg. Bake 325° for 10 to 15 minutes. Makes three muffins.

KETO COOKIES AND KETO CEREAL

2 egg whites
1 tsp. cream of tartar
1 small pkg. Sugar-free Jell-O
Beat whites stiff, add tartar and Jell-O. Pour into a nonstick pan. Bake

at 325° for 6 to 8 minutes or until brown. Makes 20 cookies.

1 serving=2 cookies.

"Cold breakfast cereal" can be made be made by adding coloring to the cookies before baking and crumbling the cookies to make cereal. Serve with allotted cream.

PEANUT BUTTER SANDWICH MEAL

4:1 345 calories
30g cream (drink)
13g cottage cheese 4%
4g Skippy peanut butter sweetener
27g egg white
26g butter
1/4 teaspoon cream of tartar

Whip whites until peaks form. Add cottage cheese, cream of tartar, and a couple drops of sweetener. Plop two piles onto cookie sheet sprayed with nonstick cooking spray. Bake at 350° for 20 to 25 minutes (until lightly brown).

To make bagels, make holes in the middle before baking. You also can fry these on a griddle. They keep nicely in the fridge. Mix butter and peanut butter together and spread on.

STRAWBERRY CHOCOLATE CHIP ICE CREAM WITH BACON

(Christopher's favorite breakfast)
Bacon
Cream
Vanilla, sweetener
Strawberries
Canola oil
Baking chocolate

Ice cream can be made up to a week beforehand: Dissolve saccharin tablet in 1/2-teaspoon of warm water. Add to cream in a small Pyrex dish. Flavor with vanilla to taste, baking chocolate shavings, and sliced fresh strawberries. Freeze about 1 hour, or until ice begins to form. Remove from freezer. Stir in canola oil quickly and return to freezer. Unmold and serve in a small bowl with crisp bacon on the side.

Options: Vary the fruit (peach, raspberry), omit the chocolate or melt it into cream, or add pure maple extract and chopped nuts for variety. Omitting chocolate or substituting chopped nuts for fruit has to be calculated, of course. Cream may be whipped before freezing.

QUICHE LORRAINE (CUSTARD WITH BACON)

Egg
Bacon
Cream
Orange

Heat cream to scald. Do not boil. Stir beaten egg into cream. Stir in crumbled bacon. Pour mixture into a custard cup. Place in a pan of water. Microwave or bake at 350° until done (about 25 minutes, or until a metal knife inserted in the middle comes out clean). Serve in the custard cup in the middle of a small plate with thin orange slices arranged around the cup in the shape of a flower.

TUNA SALAD PLATE

Tuna
Cream
Sour cream
Baking chocolate
Mayonnaise
Sugar-free Jell-O
Parmesan cheese
Cucumber, tomato, celery, lettuce

Mix mayonnaise and tuna; arrange in center of plate. Stir together sour cream and Parmesan; mix with chopped lettuce and arrange around tuna. Garnish plate with cucumbers and tomatoes. For dessert, sugarfree Jell-O topped with sweetened vanilla whipped cream, sprinkled with baking chocolate shavings.

Options: Hard-boiled egg, cubed chicken or turkey, or baby shrimps may be substituted for the tuna. These salads are easy to prepare in advance, making them ideal travel or school meals.

PEANUT BUTTER CELERY SNACKS

Celery strips
Butter

Peanut butter

Wash thin celery ribs. Peel to remove any strings. Slice off bottom for better stability. Weigh and trim. Combine peanut butter with half of allotted butter. Mix thoroughly. Fill the cavity of celery ribs with peanut butter–butter mixture. Cut into 3-inch pieces. *Note:* This menu does not have enough protein to be used as a full meal.

IN THE ABSENCE OF TOAST, *it's nice to have something crispy that holds a shape, like celery or cucumber boats. —JS*

CHEF'S SALAD WITH MAPLE WALNUT WHIP

American cheese
Lettuce, olive
Vinegar
Cream
Pure maple extract, sweetener
Ham and/or turkey
Oil
Cucumber, tomato, mushroom, carrot

Crushed walnut

Combine chopped lettuce, sliced mushrooms, and carrots in a bowl. Arrange tomato and cucumber slices, olive, and strips of cheese, ham, and/or turkey on top. Shake or beat with a fork the oil and vinegar, a speck of salt and pepper, and a few flakes of oregano in a jar with a tight lid (mayonnaise may be substituted for some of the oil for thicker consistency). Pour over salad. Sprinkle a few parsley flakes and a dash of Accent over all. For dessert: Whip cream until thick. Add 3 or 4 drops of pure maple extract and a few drops of sweetener, and continue whipping until stiff. (Several grams vegetable oil may also be whipped into cream if there is too much oil for the salad.) Heap into a parfait dish. Sprinkle with crushed walnuts and serve. Or, use butterscotch extract and chopped pecans instead for Butterscotch Fluff.

SPINACH SALAD

Hard-boiled egg

Crisp bacon
Olive oil, vinegar
Cream
Vanilla, sweetener Spinach
Mushroom, carrot, red onion
Dried mustard, garlic salt
Butter
Wash spinach, chop coarsely, place in bowl. Sprinkle with chopped red onion, sliced mushroom, and carrot. Shake oil and vinegar together in a jar with a speck of dried mustard, garlic salt, and pepper. Pour over salad. Sprinkle with crumbled crisp bacon and chopped egg (equal parts white and yolk). Serve with vanilla shake or popsicle.

AT ONE POINT MY SON STARTED GAINING WEIGHT and *I couldn't figure out why. Then Mrs. Kelly and I reviewed everything I was doing. I had started hiding a lot of fat in ice cream in the form of canola oil because my son had gotten tired of eating so much butter on top of everything. But I was measuring the oil, like the* *cream and juice, by volume. Lighter liquids are approximately equal when measured either by weight or volume. But because it is so heavy, oil has to be measured on a gram scale. When I started measuring the canola oil on the gram scale instead of in the graduated cylinder, the weight gain stopped.—JS*

DEVILED EGG WITH BERRY PARFAIT

Hard-boiled egg
Butter, mayonnaise
Grated lemon rind
Cream
Carrots, celery, onion
Dried mustard, paprika
Lettuce
Vanilla, sweetener, chocolate

Cut egg in half lengthwise and weigh equal amounts of white and yolk. Mix yolk thoroughly with mayonnaise, a few grams melted butter, a speck of dried mustard, chopped celery, and onion. Spoon yolk mixture back into the egg white. Sprinkle with salt and pepper. Dust with paprika. Serve on a plate with chopped lettuce mixed with mayonnaise and vinegar. For dessert, add vanilla and sweetener to cream and whip until stiff. Alternate whipped cream in a parfait dish with layers of sliced raspberries or strawberries.

WEIGH ALL GROUP A VEGETABLES TOGETHER, and weigh all Group B vegetables together at one time.

SHRIMP SCAMPI

Shrimp
Cream
Garlic salt Butter
Spinach

Steam shrimp and weigh. Melt butter in dish with shrimp. Add pinch of garlic salt. Steamed chopped spinach. Pat dry. Stir in some of cream if desired. Fix cream for beverage or dessert as desired.

GRILLED SALMON WITH FRESH TOMATO SALSA*

Salmon
Garlic
Green bell pepper
Cilantro
Cream
Tomato
Onion
Black olives
Olive oil

Spray pan with nonstick cooking spray; heat; season salmon with speck of salt and pepper; sear over medium to high heat until done but not dry. Remove salmon from the pan and pat dry before weighing. Meanwhile, dice tomatoes, garlic, onion, and green pepper very fine. Mix with cilantro-flavored oil (place 1g cilantro in an ounce of oil, let sit for 3 days, strain) and a speck of sea salt and pepper. Let sit for a few hours so flavors can come together. Serve salmon topped with salsa. Banana flavored ice cream for dessert.

CHICKEN SOUP AND CUSTARD

Egg
Cream
Salt (a speck)
Saccharin (1/8 grain) Diced chicken
Granulated bouillon
Carrots, celery, lettuce
Butter, mayonnaise

Custard: Scald 3 parts cream to 1 part water. Combine with 2 parts beaten egg, salt, saccharin, and vanilla. Pour into a cup and bake in a shallow pan of water 25 minutes at 350° or until done (knife inserted in center will come out clean).

Soup: Dissolve bouillon cube in 1/2-cup hot water. Add enough chicken to make up the protein left over from the egg (if any), and carrots and celery to fill the carbohydrate allotment. Melt a little butter into the soup, and spread the rest of the fat as mayonnaise on lettuce. Drink any leftover cream as beverage.

IN THE CHICKEN SOUP RECIPE, the carrots can also be made into sticks and eaten dipped in mayonnaise instead of being diced into the soup.

CREAM OF TOMATO SOUP WITH GRILLED SWORDFISH

Tomato sauce
Cream
Speck of tarragon, salt, pepper
Lettuce leaf
Celery, onion
Fresh swordfish
Mayonnaise, oil
Chocolate extract, sweetener
Sauté celery and onion in about 5g butter. Add tomato sauce. Add a speck each of tarragon, salt, and pepper. Add half of cream allotment and water to thin to desired consistency. Stir until smooth and heat until warm. Meanwhile, grill or broil seasoned swordfish, trim and weigh.

Serve with a salad of chopped lettuce mixed with mayonnaise. For dessert, put chocolate extract drops into rest of cream and pour into bowl of ice cream scoop. Chill for 1 hour. Stir in canola oil quickly and return to freezer. Freeze until hard.

FOR A VARIETY OF CREAM SOUPS, asparagus, broccoli, or spinach may be substituted for the tomato.

TREATS

BUTTER LOLLIPOPS

Soften butter. Add a tiny drop of vanilla and carbohydrate-free sweetener. Press into candy molds. Add lollipop sticks and freeze one hour or overnight. Calculate weight, not including the sticks, and serve with meals or snacks.

MACAROON COOKIES

2 egg whites
1/2 tsp. cream of tartar
1/2 package sugar-free Jell-O
Beat egg white until stiff. Add cream of tartar and dry Jell-O. Drop on aluminum foil sprayed lightly with nonstick cooking spray. Bake at 325° for 6 to 8 minutes, until brown. Cool before eating. Makes 20 cookies. One serving of two cookies contains 1.0g protein, 0g fat, 0.1g carbohydrate.

MACADAMIA BUTTERCRUNCH

Chopped macadamia nuts
Butter
Macadamia nuts are naturally in a 3:1 ratio. Add enough butter to bring them to a 4:1 ratio. This snack is good for school kids and is easy to bring along on trips.

EGGS BENEDICT*

Beaten egg
Grated cheddar cheese
Canadian bacon
Vanilla, sweetener

Cream
Butter
Cantaloupe
Scramble eggs and weigh. Place on top of heated Canadian bacon. Top with butter and cheese. Melt in broiler or microwave. Serve with cantaloupe. In a blender, blend cream with a few drops of vanilla and sweetener and two ice cubes until ice is ground into a frothy vanilla shake.

*Reproduced with permission from *The Ketogenic Cookbook* by Dennis and Cynthia Brake.

"SPAGHETTI"

Spaghetti squash
Parmesan cheese
Lettuce
Hunt's tomato sauce
Cream
Butter
Mayonnaise
Ground beef or ground turkey
Boil squash (raw squash may be frozen in individual portions in advance). Drain well and weigh. Cook

and weigh ground meat, and sprinkle on squash. Melt butter with tomato sauce and some or all of cream. Pour on top. Sprinkle grated cheese plus a speck of pepper and oregano if desired. Mix chopped lettuce with mayonnaise for a salad. Pour any remaining cream in a zero-calorie flavored soda and whip lightly for dessert.

EVEN THE SMALLEST SPRINKLE of Parmesan cheese has to be calculated into the diet. Meatballs can be frozen for later use.

HOT DOG AND CATSUP

Hebrew National hot dog
Cream cheese
Heavy cream
Catsup
Vanilla, sweetener
Butter
Zucchini or asparagus
Lettuce
Baking chocolate

Sugar-free Jell-O

Boil hot dog, drain, weigh. Mix catsup with mayonnaise to make special sauce. Cut into thin slices; dab sauce on each slice. Arrange on a small plate. Spread cream cheese (with some of the butter mixed in if desired) on lettuce. Steam vegetables; pat dry. For dessert (make in advance), add a few drops flavoring, a little sweetener, and cream to the sugar-free Jell-O. Allow to set. Or, whip cream into sweetened Jell-O and freeze in the bowl of an ice cream scoop. This is a Keto sherbet.

WHEN USING COMMERCIAL PRODUCTS such as hot dogs, the brand must always be specified. Brands of hot dog other than Hebrew National may be used in this recipe if calculations are based on accurate information about the specified brand. Jell-O desserts are often calculated into hot dog meals to raise the protein.

BROILED STEAK WITH BROCCOLI

Steak
Cream
Butter Broccoli
Mayonnaise
Broil steak to medium rare. Weigh. Steam broccoli. Melt butter, blend with mayonnaise, and pour over broccoli. Serve with cream poured into orange-flavored zero-calorie soda.

PEPPER STEAK STIR FRY AND BAVARIAN CREAM

Thin-sliced beef
Onions
Vanilla
Lettuce
Baking chocolate
Dash of soy sauce Green pepper
Mushrooms
Sweetener
Gelatin
Butter, oil
Bavarian cream: Swell 2g of gelatin with 2 tablespoons cold water. Add 2g baking chocolate and a little

of allotted butter. Place over warm water until baking chocolate, butter, and gelatin are melted. Stir in 1/4grain saccharin, a few drops vanilla, and cream. Pour into mold and freeze until hardened.

Stir fry: Heat oil equal to remaining fat allotment after butter used in Bavarian cream (some fat may be reserved for use as oil or mayonnaise in salad dressing). Sauté onions, mushrooms, and green pepper. Season with a speck of salt, pepper, and a dash of soy sauce. Cook beef separately in broiler or microwave. Weigh. Add to vegetables and serve. On the side, serve a chopped lettuce leaf with any remaining oil or mayonnaise for dressing.

IN THE BAVARIAN CREAM MEAL, total fat allotment is divided into three dishes. You can decide how much butter to melt into the Bavarian cream, how much oil to use with the stir-fry, and how much oil or mayonnaise to use as salad dressing, as long as all fats add up to the correct total.

BURGER WITH "POTATO SALAD"

Ground beef
Catsup
Salt, pepper
Cream
Vanilla, sweetener
Zucchini
Mayonnaise, oil
Oregano
Lettuce
Sugar-free Jell-O

Flatten the ground beef into a 1/4-inch thick burger. Heat a nonstick skillet with a few drops of the allotted oil or cooking spray. Sauté the burger 1 to 1-1/2 minutes on each side. Weigh the sautéed burger and trim. Meanwhile, measure the catsup and beat in an equal amount of oil. Steam zucchini. Weigh and cut into 1/2-inch cubes. Mix the zucchini with mayonnaise, oregano, and a pinch of salt and pepper. Arrange the beef on a lettuce leaf. Spread catsup mixture on steak. For dessert, top sugar-free Jell-O with whipped sweetened vanilla cream.

I BOUGHT THE KIND OF BLENDER that's a wand you can stick right into a tall glass. You just rinse the wand off in the sink after you use it. That way, I don't have to wash the whole blender every time.—FD

"PIZZA"

Egg
Tomato puree
Cream
Lettuce
Vanilla, sweetener
Olive oil
Mozzarella cheese
Pepperoni or ground beef
Speck of oregano

Beat egg with cream. Pour into heated nonstick pan. Spread thinly. Turn heat to low and let sit until hardened. Mix olive oil with tomato sauce; spread on egg crust. Sprinkle with a speck of oregano. Cover with grated cheese. Top with pepperoni or ground beef. Broil until melted. Serve with diluted cream shake. *Note:* A thin slice of eggplant, broiled, can serve as crust for alternative recipe.

21 ice cream servings. My son didn't like much *Options:* A thin tomato slice may be substituted for the egg-cream or eggplant pizza crust. Triangular slices of cheese can also make a fun pretend pizza!

BROILED FISH WITH TARTAR SAUCE

Flounder or other fish
Lettuce
Tartar sauce
Cream
Butternut squash
Sugar-free Jell-O
Butter, mayonnaise
Accent, pepper

Broil the fish about 5 minutes or until flaky. Season with a speck of Accent and pepper. Spread with measured tartar sauce. Bake butternut squash or cook frozen puree. Melt butter into squash puree. Arrange flounder on a small plate with squash and chopped lettuce with mayonnaise. Serve sugar-free Jell-O topped with whipped cream for dessert.

I DON'T COOK WITH BUTTER AS THE ALLOWED FAT. *Since the fat is his body fuel, I want him to get as much as possible. When you cook with butter, you can easily lose some of it in the pan. I usually just spray the pan with nonstick aerosol spray, cook the food, and add the butter while it's hot.—EH*

CHICKEN FINGERS AND COLE SLAW

Chicken breast
Cream
Mayonnaise
Vanilla, sweetener
Scallion
Cabbage, carrot
Butter

Heat a few drops oil in a nonstick skillet. Sauté chicken breast at medium-high heat for about 3 minutes per side or until lightly browned.

Remove chicken from heat; weigh and trim. Turn heat off. Add butter (one-third of fat allotment) to skillet. Add a dash of mustard, tarragon, and garlic salt. Stir until butter is melted. Remove skillet from heat. Cut chicken breast into thin strips or very thin slices and fan out on a small plate. Pour butter sauce over chicken. Meanwhile, chop cabbage (red or green) with a little grated carrot, thinly sliced scallion, and a leaf of lettuce. Mix mayonnaise (two-thirds of fat allotment) with a couple grams of vinegar. Stir in cabbage mixture. Sprinkle with salt and pepper. Serve with frozen vanilla-flavored cream ball.

BEEF STEW

Roast beef
Cabbage
Turnips
Baking chocolate
Pearl onions
Cherry tomatoes
Cream
Sweetener

Steam cabbage, turnip, and onion until tender. Place them in a small, nonstick pot (such as a 1-cup Pyrex) with the roast beef and 1/4 cup water. Add butter and sprinkle with a speck of salt and pepper. Simmer 15 minutes. For thicker sauce, mash some turnip into the liquid. Place cherry tomato halves around a small plate and spoon stew in center. Serve with chocolate ice cream.

CHICKEN CUTLET WITH APPLE À LA MODE

Chicken
Lettuce
Cinnamon
Apple slice
Butter/Mayonnaise
Cream
Saccharin

Chicken cutlet: Pound the chicken very thin between sheets of waxed paper. Grill or pan fry for 1 minute on each side. Sprinkle with a speck of seasoned salt or salt and pepper, and dot with some of allotted butter if desired. Spread lettuce leaf with butter or mayonnaise, roll into a pinwheel, cut in half, and arrange on small plate with chicken.

Apple à la mode: Cut center slice from a small apple. Leave skin on, remove core, and weigh. Sauté in remaining butter in a small skillet until soft. Dust with a speck of cinnamon. Place apple slice in an ice cream dish and top with a ball of sweetened vanilla frozen cream. Pour any cinnamon butter remaining in skillet on top of ice cream.

Optional: Serve with Shasta red apple diet drink.

CHICKEN WITH MASHED TURNIPS

Chicken breast
Butter
Turnips
Cream

Broil chicken breast or sauté it in a nonstick skillet with a few drops of oil. Season chicken with a few flakes of tarragon or oregano if desired. Boil turnips until soft. Mash with butter.

Season with salt and pepper. Serve with a chopped lettuce leaf and diluted cream.

CHRIS LOVED MASHED BUTTERED TURNIPS *because they reminded him of potatoes, and he loved potatoes even though he couldn't have them.—JS*

LAMB WITH CUCUMBER AND TOMATO SALAD

Lamb chop
Mayonnaise
Vinegar
Olive oil
Cucumber
Tomato
Baking chocolate
Cream

Broil lamb chop 4 minutes on each side. Season with a speck of pepper and Accent or rosemary if desired. Trim off fat and weigh lamb. Slice meat thinly and fan out on plate. Cut cucumber and tomato into 1/2-inch cubes. Combine vinegar and olive oil and pour over cucumber-tomato salad.

Serve on a chopped or rolled lettuce leaf spread with mayonnaise, with a chocolate popsicle for dessert.

"TACOS"

Ground beef
Lettuce
Cream
Chopped tomato
Grated cheese or sour cream
Speck of chili powder
Cook beef in nonstick pan. Weigh. Dust beef with a speck of chili powder. Roll beef, tomato, and cheese or sour cream in lettuce leaf. Pour cream into up to 120g of orange diet soda for a dessert drink.

EVERY WEEKEND, I WOULD MAKE 21 ice cream servings. My son didn't like much fat in his meals, so I hid almost all of it in the ice cream, which he loved and ate with every meal. I had to plan my menus in advance, so that I would know how much fat I had to hide in the ice cream for each meal. Mostly I used canola oil, which whips into the cream beautifully just before it freezes. There would be different quantities of oil whipped in with the cream, depending on each menu. Sometimes I would choose a menu with fruit and make strawberry ice cream. I had to label the ice cream very carefully as to which day and which meal they were made for. —JS

JELL-O MOLD

Sugar-free Jell-O
Cream cheese
Cream
Cottage cheese
Sour cream
Butter

Make Jell-O ahead of time and start to cool in the refrigerator. Meanwhile, whip cream. Whip in softened cream cheese, sour cream, and butter. Add 1/4g saccharin if desired. Stir into cool liquid Jell-O and let harden.

Note: This menu is helpful for children who do not chew well. Every bite is ketogenic, which means it can also be used for children during illness.

BECAUSE CREAM CONTAINS SO MUCH FAT, the more cream you use the less oil, mayonnaise, and butter you will have to fit into the rest of the menu. But if your child doesn't mind eating a lot of mayonnaise or butter, you can use less cream and fill out the carbohydrate allotment with more vegetables or fruit.

CHEESECAKE: A BIRTHDAY MEAL!

Egg
Cottage cheese
Sour cream
Cream cheese
Butter
Cream
Fruit
Vanilla, sweetener

Mix together all ingredients except fruit. Add vanilla to taste and a 1/2grain of saccharin dissolved in a 1/2-teaspoon of warm water or liquid sweetener to taste. Bake in small, greased Pyrex dish at 350° for 25 minutes or until light golden on top. Cool. Arrange fruit slices on top—sliced strawberries, pineapple, or peach. Makes a whole meal! Save a bit of cream to whip and pile on top for extra excitement.

A CHEESECAKE MEAL IS EASY TO CARRY to school in its container for special occasions, such as when other kids are eating cake to celebrate a birthday. Cheesecake also provides a ketogenic ratio in every bite, so it is useful for children who cannot eat a full meal (e.g., when recovering from an illness).

THANKSGIVING CUSTARD
Turkey breast
Turnip

Cream
Butter
Sweetener
Green beans
Canned pumpkin
Beaten egg
Speck of cinnamon
Weigh cooked turkey breast. Mash turnip with butter. Top green beans and/or turkey with rest of butter. Dessert: Whip egg, cream, canned pumpkin, dash of cinnamon, and sweetener. Bake at 325° in Pyrex dish.

Note: Cranberry sauce may be calculated into the menu, replacing both green beans and turnip.

KETOGENIC EGGNOG

Cream
Vanilla
Egg
Saccharin
Beat egg slightly. Weigh. Dissolve saccharin in 1 teaspoon or more water. Add to cream. Combine egg, cream, vanilla, and sweetener to taste.

Whip lightly if desired. Sprinkle with nutmeg. Use as travel meal or for an occasional snack. When put in the microwave, eggnog turns into a loose scrambled egg consistency.

LIKE THE CHEESECAKE, frozen eggnog in a margarine tub makes a great birthday party food. Try decorating top with fruit (strawberries, cherries). Wrap the margarine tub in colored foil and take it to school for birthday parties.

QUESTIONS ABOUT PREPARING THE DIET

Q: *Is it good to use high-fat meats to increase the fat content of the diet?*

A: Protein is very important for your child's growth. The protein portion of the diet should therefore be close to pure. Meat should be lean, trimmed of fat. Chicken and fish should be without skin. Cooked fat may be trimmed off and measured separately as part of the fat allotment for the meal. High-fat processed meats, such as sausage and bologna, should be calculated in the menu according to the manufacturer's contents.

Q: *What if some of the food sticks to the pan?*

A: Use nonstick pans and nonstick spray, and scrape out as much as possible with a small rubber spatula. Cook at low temperatures to avoid burning. Better yet, prepare food using nonstick methods: bake or broil meats, microwave eggs, steam vegetables. Remember that the allotted weights are for cooked food unless otherwise indicated, so until you are experienced with the difference between raw and cooked weights, your meats and vegetables or fruits should be prepared and cooked separately and then assembled with fats at the end.

Q: *What if my child refuses to eat the food I make?*

A: It is almost unheard of for a child to go hungry on the ketogenic diet. Remember that you are in charge, not the child! If your child has a tantrum and refuses to eat the food, give it 20 to 30 minutes, then unceremoniously throw the food out and finish the family meal. Odds are, by the next meal, your child will not be so willing to test your limits and will eat the food.

If meal battles persist, allow the child some say in choosing the food (e.g., popular choices such as hot dogs, tuna fish, etc.). Another great trick (used by pediatricians for years!) is to have your child help in the actual meal preparation (e.g., mixing mayonnaise in with tuna, counting out pieces of vegetables). Try to make the child an actual participant in the diet, not just a recipient!

Q: *Should I try to use margarine instead of butter?*

A: We recommend that you use as many unsaturated fats as possible, such as canola, safflower, flaxseed, or olive oil, or margarine made from canola oil. However, no research exists on the effect of a diet comprised of 90 percent fat, whether saturated or unsaturated. No data indicate that the ketogenic diet, despite its high fat content, leads to heart disease or atherosclerosis later in life.

Q: *My child is too disabled to care much what she eats, so I just want the simplest menu to prepare. What is easiest?*

A: The simplest ketogenic menu planning involves using the four main food groups of the diet without embellishment:

- Protein (meat, fish, chicken, cheese, egg)
- Carbohydrate (fruit or vegetable)
- Fat (butter, margarine, mayonnaise, oil)
- Cream

It takes very little time to broil a bit of meat or chicken, steam a piece of broccoli or cut up a tomato, put butter on the chicken or mayonnaise on the broccoli, and serve with a cup of cream diluted with ice and water. For a softer consistency, try fruit-topped cheesecake or custard with bacon and cooked vegetables.

Q: *What if the family has to travel, or I don't have time to prepare a meal?*

A: The eggnog recipe that you receive from your dietitian is a very good emergency or convenience food on the ketogenic diet. Chopped macadamia nuts mixed with butter can also be eaten for an occasional meal. You should not use these meals too often in the diet, but they can tide you over in a pinch. When traveling, take up to 2 days' meals ahead of time, and take them along in a portable cooler. Ask restaurants to microwave them for you if appropriate. Tuna salad with sliced vegetables such as celery, cucumbers, or carrots is especially mobile. See Chapter 6 for further details.

Q: *Can I decrease the amount of cream and use more fat in a given menu?*

A: Cream is an easy, palatable way to get a lot of fat into the diet. If desired, however, the diet can be calculated with little or no cream. The challenge will be to find ways to make a large quantity of fats or oils palatable.

CHAPTER SEVENTEEN

ATKINS DIET RECIPES

These recipes have been donated courtesy of many families who have found them helpful during their child's time on the Atkins diet. Some of these can be found on the website http://www.atkinsforseizures.com.

For other great recipe ideas, go to the Atkins approach website, www.atkins.com. Also, read Chapter 16, and use the recipes listed there for children on the ketogenic diet—just don't worry as much about portions and calories and only keep the proportions of food amounts the same.

CHOCOLATE MACADAMIA NUT MUFFINS

These look just like chocolate cupcakes

6 egg whites
6 egg yolks

1/2 tsp. cream of tartar

Liquid Sweet 'n' Low, 70 drops, divided

1/4 cup CarbSense Zero Carb Baking Mix™ (or other low-carb baking mix; soy flour will also work)

2 tsp. cocoa, sifted

1/4 cup macadamia nuts, finely chopped

1 tsp. vanilla

Frosting

4 oz cream cheese

3 T. cream, or less

3 T. unsweetened cocoa powder

1 tsp. vanilla

1/4 cup macadamia nuts, finely chopped

Separate the eggs and put the whites into mixer bowl. Add the cream of tartar and 35 drops of Sweet 'n' Low; beat until stiff peaks form. In a separate bowl, mix the egg and vanilla and beat well. Stir together the flour, cocoa, nuts, and remaining Sweet 'n'Low, add to the egg yolks and stir well. Add a good-sized spoonful of the whites to the yolks to thin the batter down. Carefully fold the batter into the egg whites, being careful not to deflate the whites.

Spray 12 muffin tins with nonstick spray, then carefully spoon the batter into them; do not flatten. Bake in a preheated 350°F to 180°C oven for 25 minutes. Remove from oven and cool on a wire rack. When cool, beat the frosting together till creamy. Spread frosting on muffins and sprinkle the nuts over top.

FRENCH TOAST

Half of a 3-ounce bag of unflavored pork rinds

Two eggs

1/4 cup heavy cream

3 packets sweetener

1/2 tsp. cinnamon

1/2 tsp. eggnog extract (optional)

Crumble pork rinds up until they resemble bread crumbs (use your food processor or put them in a Ziploc bag—with air removed—and roll them with a rolling pin.) Set aside.

Beat eggs well, and then mix with remaining ingredients and beat again.

Add crushed pork rinds to the egg/cream mixture and allow to sit for approximately 5 minutes. Mixture will thicken. Meanwhile, heat skillet or griddle with butter or oil, and when hot, fry pancake style until golden brown on both sides. Serve with your favorite zero-carbohydrate maple syrup.

Note: For the best flavor, use pork rinds with a bland taste. It's also important that you crush them well, until they are almost the texture of dust. Last, the eggnog extract is optional, but does add a nice flavor. If you don't have any, use vanilla. Recipe makes two servings.

CHEESEBURGER PIE

1 pound ground beef
scant onion powder
1 T. heavy whipping cream with enough water to make 1-1/2 cups liquid
3/4 cup Carb Sense Zero Carb Baking Mix™
3 medium eggs

1/2 tsp. salt

1/4 tsp. pepper

1 cup shredded cheese

1 T. prepared yellow mustard (optional)

In a 10-inch iron skillet, cook the hamburger and onion powder over medium heat. Break the meat up into smallish pieces with a fork and cook it until no pink shows. Drain off the fat if necessary. While the meat is cooking, in a medium sized bowl, combine the milk, baking mix, eggs, salt and pepper. Mix very well with a whisk, or combine it in a blender. It should be fairly smooth. When the meat is well cooked and drained, put it into a prepared pie plate. Top with mustard, if desired. Pour the batter over the meat. Sprinkle cheese on top. Bake the dish at 400° for about 35 minutes, longer if needed; it is puffed up and brown on top when it is done. Remove the pan from the oven and cut the meat dish into 8 wedges.

DEEP DISH PIZZA

4 ounces cream cheese, softened

2 eggs

1/4 cup Parmesan cheese, 1 ounce

1/4 tsp. oregano or Italian seasoning

1/4 tsp. garlic powder

8 ounces Italian cheese blend or mozzarella cheese, shredded

1/4 cup pizza sauce

4 ounces mozzarella cheese, shredded

Assorted toppings: pepperoni, ham, sausage, 4-ounce can mushrooms, green peppers, bacon, ground beef, etc.

Dash of garlic powder and some Italian seasoning for top of pizza

In a medium bowl, whisk cream cheese until smooth and creamy. Whisk in eggs until mixture is well-blended and smooth. Add the parmesan and seasonings, then stir in the 8 ounces of mozzarella until completely moistened. Spread cheese mixture evenly in a well-greased 9x13-inch glass baking dish. Bake at 375°F for 20 to 25 minutes or until evenly browned, but not too dark. Let cool completely on a wire rack. When nearly cooled, take a metal spatula and carefully pry up the edges to loosen from pan. Ease the spatula under the whole crust to loosen. Keep crust in the pan. This makes it easier to remove the finished pizza later. Refrigerate, uncovered, until shortly before serving time. Spread chilled crust with pizza sauce, then cheese and toppings of your choice. Lightly sprinkle with seasonings of your choice. Bake at 375°F for about 15 to 20 minutes or until toppings are bubbly. Let stand a few minutes before cutting.

FAUX FRIED RICE

Fresh head of cauliflower
1 egg
Olive oil
3 to 4 scallions
Zero-carb soy sauce
Grate one head of fresh cauliflower (or a bag of frozen and put through a food processor). *Do not use cooked*

cauliflower, because it gets too mushy. Sauté 3 or 4 green scallions in olive oil. Add the grated cauliflower. Sauté until the veggies are tender, then add a few tablespoons of zero-carb soy sauce (carefully check the label, because brands vary widely). Beat one egg and blend it into the mixture. Stir until the egg is cooked and blended into the mixture. Serve.

LEMON CAPER SALAD DRESSING

    3 T. freshly squeezed lemon juice
    1 clove garlic, minced
    2 T. capers, finely chopped
    1 T. caper juice from jar
    1/2 cup good fruity olive oil

Place garlic into processor bowl. Mince. Add capers. Mince. Add lemon juice and caper juice. Process. With processor running, add oil slowly through feed tube, blending well. This keeps well in a jar in the refrigerator for at least 2 weeks.

TURNIP FRIES

Slice and peel eight turnips as you would potatoes for fries. Place the turnips in a bowl and pour 1/2 cup of heavy cream over them. Add 10 to 20 drops of liquid Sweet 'n' Low and enough cold water to cover the turnips. Let them soak for 1/2 hour, then drain, rinse, and pat dry (this process eliminates their bitter taste). Spray a large cookie sheet heavily with baking spray. Put the following seasonings into a large plastic zippertop plastic bag: 1/4 cup Parmesan cheese, 1 tsp. Mrs. Dash Seasoning (or adobo with pepper or kosher salt), 1/4 tsp. grated nutmeg, and pepper. Shake the turnips in the bag to coat them. Spread them on the baking sheet and drizzle them with olive oil or spray them with cooking spray. Bake them in a hot 425°F oven for 15 minutes. Turn them and bake another 15 minutes. Give them a quick squirt with a slice of fresh lime before serving.

FAUX MAC AND CHEESE

One bag frozen cauliflower, cooked
3 ounces cream cheese
2 tablespoons heavy cream
1 cup shredded cheddar

Preheat oven to 350°F. Pour a little cream in bottom of baking dish and add a handful of cheddar cheese. Place cream, cream cheese, and remaining cheese in a microwave-safe dish and microwave, stirring every 30 seconds or so, until all can be stirred together easily. Pour drained cauliflower into baking dish (while cauliflower is still hot). Pour cheese mixture over and stir well to mix. Sprinkle some Parmesan over top. Bake 35 minutes; allow to stand for a few minutes before eating/serving. Recipe makes two servings as a main dish; four as a side dish.

CARB-FRIENDLY GREEK SALAD

Romaine lettuce
1/4 tsp. red wine vinegar
Sliced olives
Olive oil
Feta cheese

2–3 sliced cucumbers

PEANUT BUTTER COOKIES

1/2 cup (plus) natural creamy peanut butter

1/4 cup butter, room temperature

2 eggs

2/3 cup heavy whipping cream

1/2 tsp. baking soda

1/4 tsp. sea salt

Stevia to taste (We use about 20 drops)

Bake at 375°F for about 11 minutes.

CJ'S FRIED CHICKEN

Chicken

Egg whites

Butter

Bag of crushed pork rinds

Coconut oil

Cover the chicken in butter and egg whites, and then dip in crushed pork rinds. Fry in coconut oil. Serve.

CHOCOLATE ICE CREAM

38g 36% heavy whipping cream (whipped)

2g Hershey's unsweetened cocoa powder

1g canola oil

1g unflavored Knox gelatin

BROWNIES

4 ounces unsweetened chocolate (can be any brand as long as unsweetened)

1-1/2 sticks of butter

Bickford's vanilla flavoring, about 1-1\2 teaspoons

1 cup Splenda or NoSugar

1 cup of almond flour

3 eggs

Melt chocolate and butter together in microwave or over a pan with boiling water. Blend well. Add sugar and vanilla until well blended. Last step is to blend in eggs, then almond flour. Bake in well-greased 8x8x2 baking pan at 350°F oven for 30 to 35 minutes or until inserted toothpick comes out almost clean.

SHRIMP SCAMPI

Shelled shrimp
1/4 stick of butter
1 tsp. chopped garlic
1/4 tsp. cilantro
1/4 cup dry white wine
1/2 T. lemon juice
1 T. olive oil
Salt and pepper

Heat butter and oil over low heat, add shrimp until cooked and pink. Add garlic for 1 additional minute. Then add wine, lemon juice, salt, and pepper.

ASPARAGUS, LIMA BEAN, AND SALAMI SALAD*

8 servings, 4.5g of carbohydrates/serving

2 bunches asparagus (30 spears), trimmed and steamed (about 2 pounds)

2 T. extra-virgin olive oil

1 tsp. chopped garlic

*Recipes used with permission from Atkins.com.

1 tsp. fresh rosemary, finely chopped

1 tsp. freshly grated lemon zest (1 lemon)

3/4 tsp. salt

1/2 tsp. freshly ground black pepper

1 cup frozen baby lima beans, cooked

2 ounces Genoa salami, cut into matchstick pieces (about 2/3 cup)

In lightly salted, boiling water, cook asparagus 3 to 5 minutes, until tender-crisp. Drain into a colander and shock under cold running water for 3 minutes. Allow excess water to drain, stack in bundles and cut into 1-inch pieces. Place in a large bowl.

In the same bowl, add oil, garlic, rosemary, lemon zest, salt, and pepper.

Add lima beans and salami; toss to coat.

MINI MEXICAN PIZZA SQUARES*

10 servings, 4g of carbohydrates/serving

10 slices Atkins Bakery Country White bread™

1 cup shredded Monterey jack cheese

1/2 cup tomato salsa

2 green onions, very thinly sliced

6 black pitted black olives, sliced

2 tablespoons chopped fresh cilantro

Heat oven to 400°F. Trim crusts from bread (save to make bread crumbs). Brush bread with olive oil on one side and lightly toast.

Cut each slice into four pieces. Arrange squares on a baking sheet. Divide cheese on toast squares; top cheese with a scant tablespoon of salsa. Sprinkle with green onions and olives.

Bake 10 minutes until cheese is bubbly. Sprinkle cilantro over pizzas squares. Serve immediately.

1-1/2 T. olive oil

RASPBERRY CHEESECAKE IN A CUP*

4 servings, 5 g of carbohydrates/serving

Cheesecakes:

1 package (8 ounces) cream cheese, at room temperature

2 large eggs

1/2 cup heavy cream

3 packets Splenda™

1/4 tsp. almond extract

1/4 tsp. freshly grated lemon peel

Topping:

1/2 pint fresh raspberries

3 T. Atkins Sugar Free Raspberry Syrup™

Heat oven to 325°F. Place four 6-ounce custard cups in a large roasting pan.

Process all cheesecake ingredients in a food processor until smooth, stopping when necessary to scrape down sides of processor.

Pour batter into cups. Add enough boiling water to roasting pan to come halfway up sides of cups. Cover with foil; bake 30 minutes. Turn oven off and let stand 20 minutes. Remove from oven, uncover, and cool completely. Cover cups with plastic wrap; transfer to refrigerator to chill.

When ready to serve, toss raspberries with syrup. Evenly top cheesecakes with raspberries. Let stand at room temperature 15 minutes before serving for maximum creaminess.

CREAMY CRAB DIP (A BALTIMORE FAVORITE!)

6 servings, 1 g of carbohydrate/serving

1/4 cup mayonnaise

1/4 cup full-fat sour cream

1 tsp. Old Bay seasoning

1 tsp. fresh lemon juice

1 can (6 ounces) white crab meat, drained and picked over

2 green onions, finely chopped

2 tablespoons chopped red bell pepper

Salt

Freshly ground pepper

In a medium bowl, mix mayonnaise, sour cream, seasoning, and lemon juice until smooth. Add crab, green onions, and pepper; stir until ingredients are well combined. Season to taste with salt and pepper.

SECTION VI

SPECULATION

CHAPTER EIGHTEEN

THE FUTURE ROLE OF THE KETOGENIC DIET

The ketogenic diet presents a totally new (though actually very old) approach to the management of seizures. As we investigate and hopefully come to understand how the diet controls seizures, we may come to a new understanding of seizures and epilepsy.

Some have criticized the diet because we cannot articulate how it works. However, even modern anticonvulsant medications are usually found by serendipity. For example, valproate (Depakote) was discovered when a laboratory assistant testing compounds for anticonvulsant activity found that everything he tested was effective. He tested the solvent in which they had been placed and found that the solvent, valproic acid, was quite effective in stopping the seizures. Other new anticonvulsants are often designed to block the reuptake or to increase the production of specific neurotransmitters that excite or inhibit the firing of brain cells. While some of these "designer drugs" have been found to be effective anticonvulsants, they often work in a fashion different than that for which they were designed. Quite frankly, we do not understand epilepsy. We do not understand why a seizure occurs at a given time, what starts it, and what makes it stop. We know many of the chemical reactions that cause a single cell to fire and many of the factors that cause it to excite or inhibit the next cell in line, but epilepsy is not a problem with a single cell. A seizure is the synchronous firing of many cells causing alteration of motor function, behavior, and/or consciousness. When a problem occurs within a population of cells, it requires the proper environment and the proper conditions to fire that group of cells or a particular single cell (the focus) and to excite the surrounding cells to fire synchronously and produce a seizure. The rapidity of spread and the direction of spread determine the type of seizure. Different anticonvulsants have varied effects on the frequency and spread of different types of seizures.

One of the most remarkable things about the ketogenic diet is that, unlike most anticonvulsants, it seems to be equally effective in controlling many different types of seizures and to work on children of many different ages. Regardless of how it works, the diet appears to work by mechanisms different from most or even all chemical anticonvulsants. When we understand how the diet works, we may develop new insights into epilepsy itself, and we may be able to develop alternative mechanisms to avoid or to suppress seizures.

THINGS WE USED TO "KNOW"ABOUT KETOSIS THAT AREN'T TRUE

- *Ketosis is bad.* This misconception was based on a misunderstanding of diabetic ketoacidosis. The body's ability to utilize ketones was a survival mechanism from the time when hunter-gathers might have to go days without food in order to find game. They survived by burning their own fat stores, thus sparing muscle. Indeed, it has been calculated that a human can only survive for 3 days on stored glucose (as glycogen) but can survive up to several weeks on stored fats. Ketosis from the incomplete burning of fats is not unhealthy.

- *Fat is bad.* Our weight-conscious society has spread the misinformation that fats are bad per se, causing obesity, atherosclerosis and heart disease. They also emphasize that a low-fat diet is good. However, we have learned children on the ketogenic diet, eating a high proportion of fat for at least 2 years, have little effect on their blood lipid levels. Even the mild elevations that are found after 2 years probably disappear when the child resumes a normal, relatively low-fat diet.

- *A high-fat diet will make a person fat.* If calories ingested are limited, as is done with the ketogenic diet, a person on the diet will not gain weight. A high-fat diet, in the presence of a low number of calories, has little effect on the individual's weight. Indeed, a person can lose weight on a high-fat diet if that is a goal.

- *A high-fat diet is unhealthy and will affect growth, predispose to infection and other bad things.* These things are just not true.

Much is still to be learned about the ketogenic diet and the mechanisms of its success in controlling seizures. We will eventually learn how it works, and how we can make a diet less restrictive and perhaps even more effective. We will learn why it is dramatically effective for some children, causing their seizures to come under control within hours of the fasting alone. We will learn why, in some children, a few nuts or a small amount of glucose throws them out of ketosis and cause the return of seizures, while others have no adverse response. We will learn why some children do not respond to the diet. Is it that they do not make sufficient ketones? Is the level of ketones in the blood the critical element? Or does the seizure control have little or nothing to do with the ketone levels? Is it all due to caloric restriction?

How long must a child or an adult remain on the ketogenic diet? We do not know, and our current recommendation of 2 years is arbitrary. We have a great deal to learn about the ketogenic diet, and we can speculate that some day we will be able to package the magic ingredient of the ketogenic diet in a pill that will be equally effective and far less demanding.

SPECULATION ABOUT OTHER POSSIBLE USES OF KETOSIS AND KETOGENIC DIETS

SPECULATION means to engage in a course of reasoning based on inconclusive evidence.

Let us for a moment forget about proven uses of the ketogenic diet and speculate, on the basis of admittedly minimal and anecdotal evidence, about other areas where ketogenic diets, not necessarily the rigid ketogenic diet espoused in this book, might be of use.

- *Epilepsy in adults.* Clearly the ketogenic diet deserves study in adults with epilepsy. Small studies have suggested that it is as effective in controlling adult epilepsy as it is in children, although one study from 1930 did look at 100 adults. We are not sure why more trials have not been undertaken. One might speculate that it is because no companies would sponsor such trials and profit from their success, or that adult neurologists fear ketosis, or that physicians have been brainwashed about the bad effects of a high-fat diet. Whatever the reasons, using the ketogenic diet in adults with difficult-to-control epilepsy is clearly an area in need of study. Perhaps the Atkins diet might be of benefit in this group.

SPECULATION: The ketogenic diet will be as effective and well tolerated in adults as it is in children, and variations of the diet will in the future be used for adults with difficult-to-control epilepsy.

- *Migraine headaches.* We have heard anecdotal reports of the dramatic and long-lasting benefits of a ketogenic diet on the headaches of intractable migraine. While it has not been tested in formal studies, this might be an area worth exploring further.

SPECULATION: Variations of the ketogenic diet will be useful for those with frequent and severe migraine, particularly those who are refractory to current medications.

- *Hyperactivity, ADHD and behavior disorders.* We have seen, on occasion, dramatic improvement in the hyperactivity of children when starting the diet. Is this due to the decrease in seizures? Is it due to the decrease in medications, or is it due to some effect of the diet itself on the hyperactivity? We do not know, but this is an area that might be well worth studying.

> **SPECULATION:** Ketogenic diets may be useful in children with severe hyperactivity/attentional disorders.

- *Diabetes.* Diabetes is the inability to metabolize glucose either because of inadequate insulin production (Type 1 diabetes) or insensitivity to the insulin produced (Type 2 diabetes). If blood glucose becomes too high, the diabetic goes into what is called diabetic ketoacidosis. In this situation, the blood glucose also becomes far too high and, because the diabetic's body can't burn the glucose, it attempts to burn the body's fat. The high blood sugar causes dehydration and other chemical imbalances, and can result in death. Diabetics are given insulin to overcome their own insulin deficiency or insensitivity and thus enable them to metabolize glucose.

In the 1920s, before insulin was discovered, diabetics often survived better on a restricted glucose intake. At that time, one approach to their management was fasting for as long as was tolerated.

Because diabetic individuals can use ketone bodies derived from fat as an energy source, why not feed them a high-fat, low-carbohydrate diet, similar to the ketogenic diet? It would provide for energy needs and could be used to decrease the glucose and insulin requirements.

Ketosis also suppresses insulin production and therefore might decrease the circulating insulin and its effects on the complications of diabetes. We have corresponded with several families whose children had both diabetes and epilepsy, and who tried the ketogenic diet. We were told that these children's seizures decreased and their insulin requirements also decreased. A ketogenic diet *might* represent a new approach to the management of diabetes.

SPECULATION: Would diabetics require less insulin if fed a ketogenic diet? Probably. Would the decreased insulin requirement be beneficial? Maybe. Would this be worth carefully investigating? Definitely. A paper published in 2006 documented that a small group of Type 2 diabetic adults placed on the ketogenic diet were able to eliminate their insulin requirements, lose weight, and generally do well. More studies of the diet in the diabetic population are needed.

- *Brain tumors.* Brain tumors appear to feed on glucose. Indeed, they "steal" glucose from the surrounding brain tissue, causing the surrounding tissue to die. Whereas normal brain tissue can use ketones such as beta-hydroxy butyric acid (BOH) as an energy source, tumor tissue does not appear to have the ability to metabolize ketones.

- *Other tumors.* Leukemia cells in tissue culture die when the glucose in their media is reduced. It has been stated that these conditions would be impossible to duplicate in humans with leukemia. However, the ketogenic diet lowers blood sugar while providing sufficient energy for a normal life. Would the ketogenic diet be useful in the management of individuals with leukemia? Would it be useful in other local or systemic tumors?

SPECULATION: Would it be possible to "starve"a tumor by reducing its glucose supply, while feeding the brain with ketones? In a patient with an inoperable brain tumor that has not responded to chemotherapy, would it be reasonable to attempt a ketogenic diet, not necessarily instead of chemotherapy, but perhaps in addition to it? This is a speculation waiting to be tested.

SPECULATION: We would speculate that it is worth trying the ketogenic diet in some patients with leukemia.

Over the next decade, as the ketogenic diet becomes increasingly well accepted, as fear of a high-fat, restricted-calorie diet fades, and as fear of ketoacidosis comes into proper perspective, we speculate that the ketogenic diet, in one of its forms, will find usefulness in some of the conditions discussed here.

SECTION VII

APPENDICES

APPENDIX A

MEDICATIONS

GENERAL RULES

- Find one pharmacist who is willing to become knowledgeable about the ketogenic diet and monitor all medications and pharmaceutical products.
- Medications should be taken only in the form prescribed, since carbohydrate and sugar concentrations vary from liquids to tablets to caplets even if made by the same manufacturer.
- Ideally, your physician will order all medications from a compounding pharmacy in sugar-free or carbohydrate-free form. Locate a compounding pharmacy in your area if possible.

- In the event of emergency room treatment or hospital admission, intravenous solutions should be normal saline, not glucose or Ringer's lactated solution. Medications in a hospital setting should be given rectally or intravenously whenever possible, because these forms usually have lower carbohydrate levels.
- In the event of a life-threatening emergency, the child's immediate need for stabilization comes first. All medical personnel should be advised about the diet and advised that seizure activity may increase with glucose administration.

SOURCES OF INFORMATION

Abbott Laboratories	1-800-633-9110
Bristol-Meyers-Squibb	1-800-321-1335
Eli Lilly Laboratories	1-800-545-5979
Glaxo SmithKline	1-800-233-2426
Mead Johnson Nutritionals	1-812-429-5000
McNeil Consumer and Specialty Pharmaceuticals	1-215-273-7000
Novartis	1-888-644-8585
Pfizer	1-800-438-1985
Procter & Gamble	1-800-358-8707
Roche Laboratories	1-800-526-6367

Ross Products Division	1-800-227-5767
Roxane Laboratories	1-800-848-0120
Scot-Tussin Pharmacal Co.	1-800-638-7268
Shire US Inc.	1-800-828-2088
Teva Pharmaceuticals USA	1-800-545-8800
Wampole Laboratories	1-800-257-9525 x1
Warner-Chilcott Laboratories	1-800-424-5202
Wyeth Laboratories	1-800-544-9871

MEDICATIONS COMMONLY USED BY CHILDREN ON THE KETOGENIC DIET

The following is not intended to be a comprehensive list. Other medications may be available in each category that contain no sugar, starch, or carbohydrates and, as formulations change, some of the medications listed here may be disallowed in the future. It is important to pay close attention to labeling and to contact the manufacturer in case of doubt.

All medications on these lists contain minimal carbohydrate and may be used with the diet unless otherwise indicated.

If a medication contains less than 1g of carbohydrate per dose, it need not be calculated into the diet.

Most liquid preparations contain large amounts of sugar or sugar substitutes. Check with the manufacturer. Tablets may be a good alternative. Crushing tablets may destroy the medication in some cases, however, so check with a pharmacist if you wish to crush tablets. Children can weather most colds without the use of over-the-counter medications.

Antiepileptic medications

Carbatrol (Shire Richwood)	200mg tab=20mg lactose; 300mg tab=30mg lactose Remove from shell and use as sprinkles. Shell contains 60–90mg sugar
Depakote (Abbott)	125mg sprinkles, no carbohydrate (minute amounts of magnesium stearate in the gel capsule)
Depakote (Abbott)	125mg tab=25mg starch; 250mg tab=50mg starch; 500mg tab=100g starch
Dilantin (Parke-Davis)	30mg capsule=72mg sucrose, 74mg lactose

	100mg capsule=58mg sucrose, 74mg lactose Avoid use of Infatabs or liquid preparation
Felbamate (Wallace)	400mg tab=87mg starch, 40mg lactose
	600mg tab=130mg starch, 60mg lactose Suspension, 1,500mg=/5mLl sorbitol. Do not use.
Gabapentin (Parke-Davis)	100mg cap=14.25mg lactose, 10mg starch
	300mg cap=42.75mg lactose, 30mg starch
	400mg cap=57mg lactose, 40mg starch
Mysoline (Wyeth)	50mg tab=27.7mg lactose, 4.4mg starch
	250mg tab=22.4mg lactose, 12mg starch Suspension=.75mg/mLl saccharine sodium (this is the only sweetener)
Tegretol (Novartis)	200mg tab=51.5mg starch Avoid use of the 100mg chewable or liquid preparation.
Tegretol X-R (Novartis)	100mg tab=28mg dextrate;
	200mg tab=56mg dextrate

| Zarontin (Parke-Davis) | 250mg cap=51.1mg sorbitol Suspension=625mg/5cc sorbitol; do not use. |
| Phenobarbital (Danbury) | 30mg tabs=48mg lactose, 18mg starch |

REMEMBER: Formulations may change without notification from the manufacturer!

ANTIBIOTICS

Antibiotics commonly used by children on the ketogenic diet:

- Septra tablets (Glaxo Wellcome). Single or double strength
- Ampicillin (Squibb). 250 and 500mg. capsules
- Augmentin (SmithKline Beecham). 250mg. and 500mg. white-coated tablets or oral suspension powder (not chewable tablets or pre-mixed suspension)
- Ceclor (Lilly). 250mg. capsule (not suspension)
- Ceftin (Glaxo). 125mg., 250mg., and 500mg tablets

- Erythromycin (Abbott). 250mg. and 500mg. film-coated tablets or time-release capsule

COUGH AND COLD PREPARATIONS

Cold and cough remedies commonly used by children on the ketogenic diet:
- Benadryl Decongestant/Allergy Tablets (Parke-Davis)
- Benadryl Allergy/Sinus/Headache Tablets
- Benadryl Cold/Flu Tablets

    Benadryl Allergy contains lactose; Dye-Free Allergy contains sorbitol. Do not use.
- Comtrex Multi-Symptom Cold & Flu Tablets (Bristol Myers Squibb)
- Diabetic Tussin DM (Hi-Tech Pharmaceutical Co., Inc.). Cough suppressant/expectorant.
- Drixoral Cold & Flu Tablets,—12-Hour Formula (Schering Plough).

    Drixoral Cold & Allergy formula contains lactose and sugar. Do not use.
- Scot-Tussin DM

- Tylenol Cold Gelcaps (McNeil)
- Tylenol PM Caplets

LAXATIVES AND STOOL SOFTENERS

Constipation is a chronic problem for many children on the ketogenic diet. Laxatives, enemas, and to a lesser extent suppositories can cause dependency when used on a regular basis. Whenever possible, try to rely on less invasive measures such as stool softeners and natural bulk fiber. For any of these remedies to work effectively, sufficient fluid intake must be maintained. Be sure your child is receiving up to his full fluid allotment and offer fluids at the time of medication administration. In particularly severe cases of constipation, talk to your doctor or dietitian about increasing fluid allowances.

- Colace capsules or 1% Solution (Apothecon). Stool softener; *do not use syrup.*
- Dulcolax suppositories (CIBA Consumer)

- Fleet enema (Fleet). Use only small amount and only occasionally. Can cause dependence.
- Glycerin suppositories
- MCT oil (see p.29)
- Mineral oil. Laxative that is not absorbed by the body, but may carry essential body nutrients with it during elimination. May be used occasionally.
- Pepto-Bismol Original or Maximum Strength Liquid. Antidiarrheal. *Do not use caplets or chewable tablets.*
- Peri-Colace Capsules (Apothecon). Stool softener and laxative. Use only after you have tried regular Colace first.
- Phillips' Milk of Magnesia (original flavor only)

PAIN RELIEVERS

- Aleve Tablets
- Motrin IB Capsules (Upjohn)
- Nuprin Coated Tablets (Bristol Myers Squibb)
- Tempra (Bristol-Meyers Squibb). Infant drops; *do not use tablets or pediatric elixirs.*

- Tylenol (McNeil). Original flavor infant drops, suppositories, or regular/extra-strength tablets; *do not use pediatric elixirs.*

VITAMIN AND MINERAL SUPPLEMENTS

Liquid supplements are generally recommended for children under 1 year to 3 years of age. For older children, give one and a half to two times the dose or give supplements in tablet form. Iron preparations must be given mixed with food, because direct contact with teeth can cause black spots.

- Calcium carbonate (Rugby or Giant). 600–650mg tablets.
- Carnitor 330mg capsules; *liquid contains sugar: Do not use.*
- Fields of Nature makes many individual vitamin supplements for children with specific deficiencies.
- Lactaid Drops (McNeil Consumer Products). *Lactaid Caplets; contain mannitol: Do not use.*
- One-A-Day Essential Multi-Vitamin (tablet form for older children)
- One-A-Day Maximum Multi-Vitamin

- Poly-Vi-Sol Drops with iron; *do not give Poly-Vi-Sol in tablet form.*
- Unicap M (Multi-Vitamin in tablet form)
- Vi-Daylin Drops with iron; *do not give in tablet form.*

TOOTHPASTES AND MOUTHWASHES

- Arm & Hammer Dental Care toothpaste
- Listermint mouthwash (Warner-Lambert)
- Plax Dental Rinse—original or mint
- Scope—peppermint/mint/baking soda (Proctor & Gamble)
- Tom's of Maine toothpaste
- Ultra Brite toothpaste (Colgate-Palmolive)

MCT OIL

MCT oil can be obtained from MeadJohnson Nutritionals at a cost of approximately $65 per quart, or from Health and Sport, a distributor for Ultimate Nutrition Products. The product is called MCT Gold. It may be ordered at 1-800-305-0951. The cost is $16.00/liter plus shipping.

APPECDIX B

JOHNS HOPKINS KETOGENIC DIET ADMISSION ORDERS

 THE JOHNS HOPKINS HOSPITAL
ORDER SHEET

PEDIATRIC KETOGENIC DIET
ADMISSION ORDERS TO PEDS   *for addressograph plate*

Page 1

Ordered		Order SIGN EACH ENTRY - INCLUDE ID NUMBER *Use a ball point pen, press firmly*	Noted By	Order Completed		Initials
Date	Time			Date	Time	
		00 ADMIT/TRANSFER to PCRU				
		01 SERVICE: Neurology				
		02 ATTENDING: Dr. James Rubenstein or Dr. Eric Kossoff				
		03 RESIDENT/FELLOW:				
		04 TEAM: Zinkham or Neill				
		05 DIAGNOSIS: Intractable Epilepsy				
		06 Estimated Length of Stay: 5 Days				
		07 CONDITION: Satisfactory				
		08 VITALS: q 6 hours until tolerating 2/3 diet, then BID				
		09 D-sticks with vital signs				
		10 If blood glucose <40 with signs/symptoms of hypoglycemia, or <25 with or without signs/symptoms of hypoglycemia, give 30 cc orange juice and recheck in ½ hour. May repeat as necessary. If no results after one hour, page the pediatric neurology fellow on call				
		11 ALLERGIES:				
		12 Activity: Ad lib to playroom				
		13 MEDS: Parents to continue with home meds until seen by attending				
		14 Diet: Patient is fasting upon admission and can have only water and caffeine free, zero calorie beverages. On day _____ at _____ (meal) begin 1/3 ketogenic eggnog or formula x3 meals, 2/3 ketogenic eggnog or formula x3, then advance to full calorie ketogenic diet				
		15 Restrict fluid to _____ cc				
		16 Calories per day: _____ kcal Ratio: _____				
		17 Seizure precautions				
		18 Labs upon admission:				
		19 SIGNATURE: _____ M.D.				

Revised 2/20/03

APPENDIX C

FOOD DATABASE

CARBOHYDRATE GRAM COUNTER

Category	Code	Description	Grams	Protein	Fat	Carb	Kcal
BABY	BAPAP	Gerber Apple/ Apricot	100	0.22	0.22	11.63	49
	BAPPA	Gerber Apple/ Pineapple	100	0.08	0.08	10.08	41
	BAPPL	Strained Apples	100	0.16	0.16	10.94	46
	BAPRA	Gerber Apple/ Raspberry	100	0.22	0.15	15.17	63
	BBATA	Gerber Banana Tapioca	100	0.37	0.07	15.26	63
	BBEEF	Strained Beef	100	13.64	5.35	0	103
	BBEET	Strained Beets	100	1.33	0.08	7.66	37
	BCARR	Strained Carrots	100	0.78	0.16	6.02	29
	BCHIC	Strained Chicken	100	13.74	7.88	0.1	126

	BGRBE	Strained Green Beans	100	1.33	0.08	5.94	30
	BLAMB	Strained Lamb	100	14.04	4.75	0.1	99
	BMIXV	Strained Mixed Vegeta-bles	100	1.25	0.47	7.97	41
	BPEAC	Strained Peaches	100	0.52	0.15	18.89	79
	BPEAR	Strained Pears	100	0.31	0.16	10.86	46
	BPEAS	Strained Peas	100	3.52	0.31	8.13	49
	BPEPA	Strained Pear/ Pineapple	100	0.31	0.08	10.86	45
	BSQUA	Strained Squash	100	0.86	0.16	5.63	27
	BTURK	Strained Turkey	100	15.35	7.07	0	125
	BAPBL	Gerber Apple/ Blueberry	100	0.22	0.22	16.3	68
DAIRY	CHAM	American Cheese	100	19.05	23.81	9.52	329
	CHCH	Cheddar Cheese	100	21.43	32.14	3.57	389
	CHCO	Cottage Cheese, 2% Low-fat	100	13.16	2.19	2.63	83

	CHCR	Cream Cheese, Philadel-phia Brand	100	6.67	33.33	3.33	340
	CHMON	Monterey Cheese	100	24.64	30.71	0.71	378
	CHMOZ	Mozzarel-la Cheese, Whole Milk	100	21.43	25	3.57	325
	CHPAR	Parme-san, Grat-ed	100	42	30	4	454
	CHSW	Swiss Cheese	100	24.5	24.85	2.1	332
	CHWZ	Cheez Whiz, Kraft	100	16.43	20.36	6.43	275
	CREA1	Cream, 36%	100	2	36	3	344
	CREA2	Cream 30%	100	2	30.67	2.67	295
	EGG	Egg, Fresh	100	12	9	1.2	134
	SOUR	Sour Cream	100	3.33	16.67	6.67	190
	YOGUR	Yogurt, Plain Low-fat	100	5.24	1.54	7.05	63

			100				
	CHMOZ2	Mozzarella Cheese, Part Skim	100	28.57	17.86	3.57	289
	CHCO2	Cottage Cheese 4% Low-fat	100	13.16	4.39	3.51	106
	CHRC	Ricotta Cheese, Whole Milk	100	9.68	12.9	6.45	181
	CHRC2	Ricotta Cheese, Part Skim	100	10.34	7.76	6.9	139
	WHMK	Whole Milk (ML)	100	3.39	3.39	5.02	64
FATS	BUTT	Butter	100	0.67	81.33	0.00	735
	MARG	Margarine, Stick Corn	100	0.00	76	0.00	684
	MAYO	Mayonnaise, Hellman	100	1.43	80	0.7	729
	OILC	Corn Oil	100	0.00	97.14	0.00	874
	OILO	Olive Oil	100	0.00	96.43	0.00	868
	OILP	Puritan Oil	100	0.00	100	0.00	900
	OILM	MCT Oil	100	0.00	92.67	0.00	834
FISH	FLOU	Flounder, Baked	100	24.12	1.53	0.00	110
	HADD	Haddock, Baked	100	24.3	0.95	0.00	106

	LOBST	Lobster, Raw	100	18.82	0.94	0.47	86
	REDS	Red Snapper, Raw	100	26.35	1.76	0.00	121
	SALM	Salmon, Raw	100	20	3.41	0.00	111
	SCAL	Scallops, Raw	100	16.82	0.71	2.35	83
	SHRIM	Shrimp, Raw	100	20.35	1.76	0.94	101
	SWORD	Swordfish, Baked	100	25.41	5.18	0.00	148
	TROUT	Rainbow Trout	100	26.35	4.35	0.00	145
	TUNA1	Tuna Lt Chnk StarKist/Oil	100	22.41	22.41	0.00	291
	TUNA2	Tuna Lt Chnk StarKist/Water	100	23.21	0.89	0.00	101
	TUNA3	Tuna All White StarKist/Water	100	21.43	8.93	0.00	166
	TUNA4	Tuna, Fresh	100	29.88	6.24	0.00	175
FRUIT	APPLE	Apple	100	0.21	0.36	14.84	63

	APPLS	Apple-sauce, Unsweet-ened	100	0.16	0.08	11.31	47
	APRI	Apricot	100	1.42	0.38	11.13	54
	BANAN	Banana	100	1.05	0.53	23.42	103
	BLUE	Blueber-ries	100	0.69	0.41	14.14	63
	CANT	Can-taloupe	100	0.88	0.25	8.38	39
	CHERR	Cherries	100	1.18	1.03	16.62	80
	FRCOC	Fruit Cocktail Canned/ Water	100	0.41	0.08	8.52	36
	GRAFR	Grape-fruit, Pink	100	0.57	0.08	7.72	34
	GRAPG	Green Grapes	100	0.65	0.33	17.17	74
	GRAPP	Purple Grapes	100	0.69	0.56	17.75	79
	HONML	Honey-dew Mel-on	100	0.8	0.3	7.7	37
	JAPP	Apple Juice	100	0.1	0.1	11.7	48
	JORAN	Orange Juice	100	0.7	0.2	10.4	46
	LEMON	Lemon	100	1.03	0.34	9.31	44
	LEMRI	Lemon Rind	100	1.67	0.00	16.67	73

			100				
	MAN-GO	Mango	100	0.53	0.29	17	73
	NECT	Nectarine	100	0.96	0.44	11.76	55
	ORANG	Orange, Navel	100	1	0.07	11.64	51
	PEACH	Peach	100	0.69	0.11	11.15	48
	PEAR	Pear	100	0.42	0.42	15.12	66
	PINEA	Pineapple	100	0.39	0.45	12.39	55
	PLUM	Plum	100	0.76	0.61	13.03	61
	PUMPK	Pumpkin, Canned	100	1.07	0.25	8.11	39
	RASP	Raspber-ries	100	0.89	0.57	11.54	55
	STRAW	Strawber-ries	100	0.6	0.4	7.05	34
	TANG	Tangerine	100	0.6	0.24	11.19	49
	WATML	Watermel-on	100	0.63	0.44	7.19	35
GENER-IC	GMFP	Generic Meat, Fish, Poul-try	100	23.3	16.7	0.00	243
	GFRU	Generic 10% Fruit Exchange	100	1	0.00	10	44
	GVEG	Group B Vegetable Exchange	100	2	0.00	7	36
	GPBUT	Generic Peanut Butter	100	26	48	22	624

	GFAT	Butter, Mar-garine, Mayo	100	0	74	0.00	666
	GSTMT	Generic Strained Meats	100	13.33	6.67	0.00	113
MEAT	BACO	Bacon, Oscar Mayer	100	33.33	41.67	0.00	508
	BEEF1	Eye Round Beef	100	29	6.5	0.00	175
	BEEF2	Lean Ground Beef Medi-um	100	24.2	19.1	0.00	269
	BOLO1	Beef Bologna, Oscar Mayer	100	10.71	28.57	3.57	314
	BOLO2	Beef Bologna, Hebrew National	100	10.71	10.71	2.86	151
	CAN-BAC	Canadian Bacon, Oscar Mayer	100	19.58	4.17	0.42	118

Cate-gory	Code	De-scrip-tion	Grams	Pro-tein	Fat	Carb	Kcal
	CORBF	Corned Beef, Oscar May-er	100	20	1.76	0.59	98
	HAM	Cured Ham, Cen-ter Slice	100	20.2	12.9	0.1	197
	HOTD1	Beef Frank, He-brew Na-tional	100	12.5	29.17	2.08	321
	HOTD2	Beef Frank Oscar May-er	100	11.11	28.89	2.22	313
	LAMB	Leg of Lamb, Lean	100	28.71	7.06	0	178
	LEAN	Lean and Tasty	100	23.3	35.8	0.8	419
	PORK	Pork Chop, Lean Broiled	100	32	10.5	0	223

	SAUS1	Oscar Mayer Pork, Beef Link	100	13.3	27.8	2.2	312
	SAUS2	Sausage, Bob Evans	100	13.57	30.71	2.5	341
	SAUS3	Sausage, Hillshire Farm	100	12.28	29.82	3.51	332
	VEAL	Veal Cutlet	100	27.06	11.06	0	208
MISC	CHOC1	Baking Chocolate, Bakers	100	11.07	52.14	30	634
	CHOC2	Baking Chocolate, Hershey's	100	14.29	56.43	23.93	661
	CO-COA	Hershey's Cocoa	100	27.3	12.8	45.7	407

	JEL-LO	Jell-O Sugar-Free Gelatin	100	1.16	0	0.17	5
	MUST1	Mus-tard Yel-low	100	4	4	6	76
	OLIV1	Olives, Green	100	1.09	10.65	1.09	105
	OLIV2	Olives, Black	100	1.67	28.75	7.08	294
	SOY	Soy Sauce	100	10.52	0.17	5.52	66
	TAR-TA	Tar-tar Sauce, Kraft	100	0	64.29	0	579
	VINEG	Vine-gar, Dis-tilled	100	0	0	5.33	21
NUTS	AL-MON	Al-monds, Dry Roast-ed	100	16.43	52.5	24.64	637
	BRAZ	Brazil Nuts	100	14.64	67.14	12.86	714

CASH	Cashews, Dry Roast-ed	100	15.71	47.14	34.29	624
MACAD	Macadamia Nuts	100	8.57	75.71	8.93	751
PEAN1	Peanuts, Dry Roast-ed	100	23.57	49.64	21.43	627
PEAN2	Peanuts, Oil Roast-ed	100	29.64	48.57	16.07	620
PECAN	Pecans	100	8.21	65.71	22.5	714
PETE	Peter Pan Chunky Peanut But-ter	100	25	50	22	638
PIST	Pista-chio Nuts	100	15	53.57	27.86	654
SKIP	Skip-py Creamy Peanut But-ter	100	28.13	53.13	15.6	653
SUNF	Sun-flow-er Seeds	100	23.21	50.36	18.93	622

	WALN	Walnuts, Black, Dried	100	24.64	57.5	12.14	665
POULTRY	CHIC	Chicken Breast — No Skin (Cooked)	100	31.05	3.6	0	157
	TURK	Turkey Breast	100	29.9	3.2	0	148
SOUP	BOUL1	Wylers Inst Boull — Chicken/Beef	100 0.00	0	28.57	114	
	BROTH1	Swanson Canned — Chicken (ML)	100 0.83	0.83	0.42	12	
	BROTH2	Swanson Canned — Beef (ML)	100	0.83	0.42	0.42	9

			100	0	10.42	1.25	9
	BROTHB	Swanson Canned — Vegetable (ML)	100	0	10.42	1.25	9
TUBE	TMI-CR	Microlipid (ML)	100	0	50	0	450
	TPLOY	Poly-cose Powder	100	0	0	94	376
	TR-CFC	RCF Concentration (ML)	100	4	7.2	0	81
VEG-ETABLE	AS-PAR	Asparagus — C (Grp A)	100	2.56	0.33	4.44	31
	BEAN1	Green Beans	100	1.94	0.32	7.9	42
	BEET	Beets — C (Grp B)	100	1.06	0	6.71	31

BROC	Broc-coli — C (Grp B)	100	2.95	0.25	5.5	36
BRUS	Brus-sels Sprouts	100	2.56	0.51	8.31	48
CABB1	Cab-bage, Green — R	100	1.14	0.29	5.43	29
CABB2	Cab-bage, Green — C	100	0.93	0.13	4.8	24
CARR	Car-rots — R or C (Grp B)	100	1.15	0.13	10.5	48
CATS	Toma-to Cat-sup	100	2	0.67	25.33	115
CAUL	Caulflow-er — C (Grp B)	100	2	0.2	5	30

	CELE	Cel-ery — R or C (Grp A)	100	0.75	0.25	3.75	20
	CHIVE	Chives — R	100	3.33	0	3.33	27
	CORN	Corn, Yel-low	100	3.29	1.34	25.12	126
	CUCU	Cu-cum-ber — R (Grp A)	100	0.58	0.2	2.9	16
	EGG-PL	Egg-plant — C (Grp A)	100	1.22	0	6.34	30
	EN-DIV	En-dive	100	1.2	0.4	3.2	21
	KALE	Kale — C (Grp B)	100	1.85	0.46	5.69	34
	LETT	Let-tuce, Ice-berg (Grp A)	100	1	0	2	12

	MUSH1	Mush-rooms — R	100	2	0.57	4.57	31
	MUSH2	Mush-rooms, Canned	100	1.92	0.26	5	30
	MUST	Mus-tard Greens — C	100	2.29	0.29	2.14	20
	OKRA	Okra — C (Grp B)	100	1.88	0.13	7.25	40
	ONION	Onions, Raw	100	1.13	0.25	7.38	36
	PARSL	Pars-ley — R	100	2.33	0.33	7	40
	PEAS	Green Pea — R	100	5.38	0.38	14.49	83
	PEPP	Green Pep-pers — R or C (Grp A)	100	0.8	0.4	5.4	28
	PICK	Dill Pickle Slices	100	0.8	0	2.3	12

	POTA1	Pota-to — Boiled w/ o Skin	100	1.7	0.07	20	87
	POTA2	Pota-to — Baked w/ Skin	100	2.33	0.1	25.25	111
	RADI	Radish — R (Grp A)	100	0.67	0.44	3.56	21
	SAUER	Sauerkraut — C (Grp A)	100	0.93	0.17	4.32	23
	SPIN1	Spinach — R	100	2.86	0.36	3.57	29
	SPIN2	Spinach, Frozen, w/Butter, Pills-bury	100	3	1	4.4	39
	SPROU	Bean Sprouts, Mung — R	100	3.08	0.19	5.96	38
	SQUAS	Spaghetti Squash	100	0.64	0.26	6.41	31

	TOMA	Toma-to, Red — R	100	0.89	0.24	4.31	23
	TOMAC	Toma-to, Canned in Puree	100	0.84	0.84	5.04	31
	TOMAP	Toma-to Paste, Canned	100	3.82	0.92	18.85	99
	TOM-PU	Toma-to Puree	100	1.68	0.12	10.04	48
	TOM-SA	Spaghetti Sauce w/Meat	100	2.12	5.13	17.88	126
	TURNI	Turnips, Boiled	100	0.77	0.13	4.87	24
	ZUCCH	Zuc-chini — C (Grp A)	100	1.23	0.15	2.92	18

APPENDIX D

ATKINS CARBOHYDRATE GRAM COUNTER

FOOD	CARBOHYDRATE GRAMS
MILK PRODUCTS	
Cream (light, 1tbsp)	0.6
Cream (sour, 2tbsp)	1.0
Cream (heavy, 1tbsp)	0.5
Half and Half (1tbsp)	0.7
Milk (whole, 1cup)	11.0
Milk (soy, unsweetened, 1cup)	13.0
Plain Yogurt (skim, 1cup)	13.0
(whole,1 cup)	12.0

FOOD	CARBOHYDRATE GRAMS
CHEESE	
American (1 oz)	0.5
Camembert (1 oz)	0.5
Cheddar (1 oz)	0.6
Cottage (fat-free, 1 cup)	10.0
Cottage (whole, 1 cup)	8.0
Cream Cheese (2 tbsp)	1.0
Feta (1 oz)	1.0

Muenster (1 oz)	1.0
Provolone (1 oz)	1.0
Swiss (1 oz)	0.5

FOOD	CARBOHYDRATE GRAMS
NUTS	
Almond Paste (1 oz)	14.5
Almonds (1 oz)	5.5
Brazil (1 oz)	3.1
Cashews (1 oz)	8.3
Coconut (1 oz)	4.3
Hazelnuts (filberts) (1 oz)	4.7
Macadamia (1 oz)	4.5
Peanut Butter (1 tbsp)	3.0
Peanuts (1 oz)	5.4
Pecans (1 oz)	4.1
Pignolia (1 oz)	3.3
Pistachio (1 oz)	5.4
Pumpkin Seeds (1 oz)	4.2
Sesame Seeds (1 tbsp)	1.4
Soybeans (1.2 cup)	6.0
Sunflower Seeds (1 oz)	5.6
Walnuts (1 oz)	4.2

FOOD	CARBOHYDRATE GRAMS
GRAINS	
Bagel (1)	30.0

Bread (pumpernickel, 1 slice)	17.0
Bread (whole wheat, 1 slice)	11.0
Corn Muffin	20.0
Farina (1 cup)	22.0
Frozen Waffle	29.0
Noodles (1 cup cooked)	37.3
Oatmeal (1 cup cooked)	27.0
Pancake (using dry mix)	17.4
Popcorn (popped 1 cup)	5.0
Rice (cooked 1 cup)	49.6
Rice (puffed 1 cup)	11.5
Pancake (using dry mix)	17.4
Popcorn (popped 1 cup)	5.0
Rice (cooked 1 cup)	49.6
Rice (puffed 1 cup)	11.5

FOOD	CARBOHYDRATE GRAMS
SOUPS	
Chicken Consommé (1 cup)	1.9
Chicken Gumbo (1 cup)	7.4
Cream of Chicken (1 cup)	14.5
Cream of Mushroom (1 cup)	16.2
Turkey Rice (1 cup)	10.0

FOOD	CARBOHYDRATE GRAMS
HERBS	
Allspice (1 tsp)	1.4
Basil (1 tsp)	0.9
Caraway (1 tsp)	1.1
Celery (1 tsp)	0.6
Cinnamon (1 tsp)	1.8
Coriander Leaf (1 tsp)	0.3
Dill Seed (1 tsp)	1.2
Garlic Clove (1)	0.9
Ginger Root (fresh, 1 oz)	3.6
Ginger Root (ground, 1 tsp)	1.3
Saffron (1 tsp)	0.5
Tarragon (1 tsp)	0.8
Thyme (1 tsp)	0.9
Vanilla (double strength, 1 tsp)	3.0

FOOD	CARBOHYDRATE GRAMS
VEGETABLES	
Asparagus (4 spears)	2.2
Beans, green (boiled, 1 cup)	6.8
Beans, yellow or wax (boiled, 1 cup)	5.8
Broccoli (1 cup)	8.5
Brussels Sprouts (1 cup)	9.9

Cabbage (1 cup)	6.2
Carrot (7 in.)	7.0
Cauliflower (1cup)	5.1
Celery (1 stalk)	1.6
Coleslaw (1 cup)	8.5
Collards (1 cup)	9.8
Corn (1 ear, 5 in.)	16.2
Cucumber (sliced, 1 cup)	3.6
Dandelion (1 cup)	6.7
Endive (1 cup)	2.1
Kale (1 cup)	6.7
Kohlrabi (1 cup)	8.7
Lettuce (Romaine, 1 cup)	1.9
Lettuce (Boston, 1 cup)	1.4
Lettuce (Iceberg, 1 cup)	1.6
Mushrooms (1 cup)	3.1
Mustard Greens (1 cup)	5.6
Okra (1 cup)	9.6
Onion (1 cup)	14.8
Parsley (1 tbsp)	0.3
Parsnips (1 cup)	23.1
Peas (1 cup cooked)	19.4
Peppers (green, 1 cup)	7.2
Peppers (red, dried, 1 tsp)	1.4
Potato (baked, 1)	32.8
Potato Salad (1 cup)	33.5
Pumpkin (31.2 oz)	7

Radish (large, 10)	2.9
Spinach (1 cup)	6.5
Squash (summer, 1 cup)	6.5
Squash (winter, 1 cup)	25.5
Sweet Potato (baked, 1)	37.0
Tomato (raw 21.2 in.)	5.8
Tomato (cooked, 1 cup)	13.3
Tomato (juice, 1 cup)	10.4
Turnips (cooked, 1 cup)	11.3
Turnips (greens, 1 cup)	5.2

FOOD	CARBOHYDRATE GRAMS
PROTEIN (FAT OR LEAN, WITHOUT BREADING)	
Fish, Poultry, Meat or Eggs	0-trace

FOOD	CARBOHYDRATE GRAMS
FATS/OILS	
Olive, Canola, Safflower, etc.	0-trace

FOOD	CARBOHYDRATE GRAMS
BEANS	
Black-eyed (1 cup)	38
Lima (1 cup)	33.7
Navy (1 cup)	40.3
Red Kidney (1 cup)	39.6

Soybeans (1 cup cooked)	19.4
Split Peas (1 cup)	41.6
Tofu/Bean Curd (2-in. cube)	2.9

FOOD	CARBOHYDRATE GRAMS
FRUIT	
Apple (1 medium, 23.4 in.)	20
Applesauce (unsweetened, 1 cup)	26.4
Apricots (fresh, 3)	13.7
Avocado (California)	13.0
Avocado (Florida)	27.0
Banana (1)	26.4
Blackberries (1 cup)	18.6
Blueberries (1 cup)	22.2
Cantaloupe (1.2 melon, 5 in.)	20.4
Cherries (1 cup)	20.4
Grapefruit (pink, 1.2)	10.3
Grapes (10)	9.0
Honeydew (1 cup)	13.1
Kiwi (1 medium)	9
Lemon	6.0
Lemon Juice (1 cup)	19.5
Mango (1 cup)	27.7
Olive (green, pitted)	2.5
Orange (1 medium)	16.0

Papaya (1 medium)	30.4
Peach (21.2 in.)	9.7
Pear (31.2 in.)	31.0
Pineapple (1 cup)	21.2
Plum (1 medium)	17.8
Prunes (1)	5.6
Raspberries (1 cup)	21
Rhubarb (cooked w/sugar, 1 cup)	97.2
Strawberries (1 cup)	12.5

FOOD	CARBOHYDRATE GRAMS
SAMPLES OF CARBOHY-DRATE "FATTENING"ITEMS	
Apple Pie (homemade, 1 slice)	61
Apple Turnover	30
Banana Split	91
Bean Burrito	48
Cheeseburger (1.4 pounder)	33
Chicken Salad Sandwich	27
Cornbread Stuffing (1.2 cup)	69
Devil Dog	30
Egg Roll (1)	30
French Toast (2 slices)	34
Graham Crackers (1)	5

(chocolate covered, 1)	8
Hard Candy, Gumdrops, Jelly Beans (1 oz)	25
Honey (1 oz)	34
Hot Dog with Bun (1)	24
Ice Cream Soda (1 cup)	49
Macaroni with Cheese (1 cup)	40
Onion Rings (fast food order)	33
Peanut Brittle (1 oz)	23
Pecan Pie (homemade, 1 slice)	41
Pizza (1 slice)	24
Popsicle	17
Rolled Oats (1 cup cooked)	23
Saltines (1)	2
Shake (medium)	90
Sherbet (lemon, 1.2 cup)	45
Soda Crackers (1)	4
Tapioca Cream (1.2 cup)	22
Toaster Pastry (frosted, blueberry)	34
Waffles (plain, homemade, 1)	28
Whaler	64
White Sugar (1 oz)	28

APPENDIX E

USEFUL WEBSITE

ORGANIZATIONS

http://www.neuro.jhmi.edu/Epilepsy/Peds

Johns Hopkins Pediatric Neurology website, with information about the ketogenic diet, the Atkins diet, and international keto-genic diet centers

http://www.charliefoundation.org

The Charlie Foundation to Help Cure Pediatric Epilepsy

http://www.atkinsforseizures.com

A useful website created by the family of a child in the first Hopkinspediatric Atkins study

http://www.atkins.com

Recipes and advice on the Atkins diet

http://www.shsweb.co.uk/neuro/ketocal.htm

Information about KetoCal™, a ketogenic diet formula supplement

http://www.epilepsyfoundation.org

The Epilepsy Foundation website
http://www.aesnet.org
American Epilepsy Society website
http://www.epilepsy.com
General information about epilepsy sponsored by the Epilepsy Therapy Development Project
http://www.ilae.org
International League Against Epilepsy website
http://www.lowcarb.ca
Website with support, information, and recipes for low-carb dieters

PRODUCT INFORMATION

http://www.specialcheese.com/bakedch.htm
Just the Cheese™ snacks
http://www.dukesmayo.com
High-fat, sugar-free mayonnaise
http://www.kraftfoods.com/fruit2o
Information about Fruit2O™ products
http://www.bickfordflavors.com
No-carbohydrate flavorings
http://www.tomsofmaine.com

No-carbohydrate toothpaste
http://www.carbsense.com

Makers of low-carb products with plenty of fiber
http://www.calorieking.com

Information about *The 2005 Doctor's Pocket Calorie, Fat & Carb Counter,* a helpful resource for Atkins patients

APPENDIX F

SELECTED REFERENCES

GENERAL INFORMATION ON EPILEPSY

Freeman JM, Vining EPG, and Pillas DJ. *Seizures and Epilepsy: A Guide for Parents.* Baltimore: Johns Hopkins University Press, 2001.

RECENT REFERENCES ON THE EFFECTIVENESS AND ACCEPTABILITY OF THE KETOGENIC DIET

Freeman JM, Vining EPG. Seizures rapidly decrease after fasting: preliminary studies of the ketogenic diet. *Arch Pediatr Adolesc* 1999; 153; 946–949.

Freeman JM, Vining EPG, Pillas DJ, Pyzik PL, Casey JC, Kelly MT. The efficacy of the ketogenic diet—1998: a prospective evaluation of intervention in 150 children. *Pediatrics* 1998; 102: 1358–1363.

Nordli DR, Jr., Kurodamm, Carroll J, et. al. Experience with the ketogenic diet in infants. *Pediatrics* 2001; 108: 129-33.

Rubenstein JE, Kossoff EH, Pyzik PL, Vining EPG, McGrogan JR, Freeman JM. Experience in the use of the ketogenic diet as early therapy. *J Child Neurol* 2005; 20: 31-4.

Gilbert DL, Pyzik PL, Vining EPG, Freeman JM. Medication cost reduction in children on the ketogenic diet: data from a prospective study of 150 children over one year. *J Child Neurol* 1999; 14: 469–471.

Hemingway C, Freeman JM, Pillas DJ, Pyzik PL. The Ketogenic Diet: A 3-to 6-year follow-up of 150 children enrolled prospectively. *Pediatrics* 2001; 108: 898–905.

Kim DW, Kang HC, Park JC, Kim HD. Benefits of the nonfasting ketogenic diet compared with the initial fasting ketogenic diet. *Pediatrics* 2004; 114: 1627–30.

Kossoff EH. More fat and fewer seizures: Dietary therapy for epilepsy. *Lancet Neurol* 2004; 3: 415–20.

Kossoff EH, McGrogan JR. Worldwide use of the ketogenic diet. *Epilepsia* 2005; 46: 280-9.

Kossoff EH, Krauss GL, McGrogan JR, Freeman JM. Efficacy of the Atkins Diet as therapy for intractable epilepsy. *Neurology* 2003; 61: 1789–91.

Kossoff EH, Pyzik PL, McGrogan JR, Vining EPG, Freeman JM. Efficacy of the ketogenic diet for infantile spasms. *Pediatrics* 2002; 109: 780–3.

LeFevre F, Aronson N. Ketogenic diet for the treatment of refractory epilepsy in children: a systematic review of efficacy. *Pediatrics* 2000; 105(4) (Abstract).

Mady MA, Kossoff EH, McGregor AL, Wheless JW, Pyzik PL, Freeman JM. The Ketogenic Diet: Adolescents Can Do It, Too. *Epilepsia* 2003; 44: 847–51.

Swink TD, Vining EPG, Freeman JM, The ketogenic diet 1996, *Adv Pediatr* 1997; 44: 297–329.

Than KD, Kossoff EH, Rubenstein JE, Pyzik PL, McGrogan JR, Vining EPG. Can you predict an immediate, complete, and sustained response to the ketogenic diet? *Epilepsia* 2005; 46: 580–2.

Vining EPG, Freeman JM, for the Ketogenic Diet Study Group. A multi-center study of the efficacy of the ketogenic diet. *Arch Neurol* 1998; 55: 1433–37.

Wheless JW. The Ketogenic Diet: An effective medical therapy with side effects. *J Child Neurol* 2001; 16: 633–35.

OTHER BOOKS OF INTEREST

Keith, Haddow M. *Convulsive Disorders in Children: With Reference to Treatment with the Ketogenic Diet.* Boston: Little, Brown and Company, 1963; Chapters 12 & 13.

Lennox, William G. *Epilepsy and Related Disorders.* Boston: Little, Brown and Company, 1960. Vol 2: 734–39, 824–32.

Livingston, S. *Living with Epileptic Seizures.* Springfield, Ill.: Charles C. Thomas, 1963: 143–63.

Livingston, Samuel. *The Diagnosis and Treatment of Convulsive Disorders in Children.* Springfield, Ill.: Charles C. Thomas, 1954: 213–36.

Stafstrom, Carl, Rho, Jong, editors. *Epilepsy and the Ketogenic Diet.* Totowa, N.J.: Humana Press, 2004.

THE MEDIUM-CHAIN TRIGLYCERIDE (MCT) DIET

Atkins, Robert C. *Dr. Atkins' New Diet Revolution.* New York: Avon, 2002.

Huttenlocher PR, Wilbourn AJ, Signore JM. Medium-chain triglycerides as a therapy for intractable epilepsy. *Neurology* 1971; 21: 1097–1103.

Sills MA, Forsyth WI, Haidukwych D. The medium-chain triglyceride diet and intractable epilepsy. *Arch Disease in Childhood* 1986: 1169–72.

Trauner, DA. Medium-chain triglyceride (MCT) diet in intractable seizure disorders. *Neurology* 1985: 237–38.

OTHER ARTICLES OF INTEREST

Casey JC, Vining EPG, Freeman JM, et al. The implementation and maintenance of the ketogenic diet in children. *J Neurosci Nurs* 1999; 31: 294–302.

De Vivo DC, Pagliara AS, Prensky AL. Ketotic hypoglycemia and the ketogenic diet. *Neurology* 1973; 23: 640–49.

Dodson WE, Prensky AL, De Vivo DC, Goldring S, Dodge PR. Management of seizure disorders: selected aspects. Part II. *J Pediatr* 1976; 89: 695–703.

Herzberg GZ, Fivush BA, Kinsman SL, Gearhart JP. Urolithiasis associated with the ketogenic diet. *J Pediatr* 1990; 117: 743–45.

Livingston S, Pauli S, Pruce I. Ketogenic diet in the treatment of childhood epilepsy. *Dev Med Child Neurol* 1977; 19: 833–34.

Millichap JG, Jones JD, Rudis BP. Mechanism of anticonvulsant action of ketogenic diet. *Am J Dis Child* 1964; 107: 593–603.

Schwartzkroin PA. Mechanisms underlying the anti-epileptic efficacy of the ketogenic diet. *Epilepsy Res* 1999; 37: 171–80.

Stafstrom CE. Animal models of the ketogenic diet: what have we learned, what can we learn? *Epilepsy Res* 1999; 37: 241–59.

Withrow CD. Antiepileptic drugs. The ketogenic diet: mechanism of anticonvulsant action. In: Glaser GH, Penry JK, Woodbury DM, eds. *Antiepileptic Drugs: Mechanisms of Action.* New York: Raven Press, 1980: 635–42.

APPENDIX G

INTERNATIONAL CENTERS

This is a partial list of centers around the world that offer the ketogenic diet (and have relatively good e-mail contact). This does not represent all centers in the world and is by no means an endorsement of their ketogenic diet programs. For an updated list, go to http://www.neuro.jhmi.edu/E pilepsy/Peds/ketoworldwide.htm.

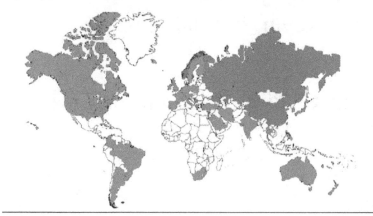

This map has been reproduced with permission from *Epilepsia*.

NORTH AMERICA

Drs. Peter and Carol Camfield

Dalhousie University and the
IWK Grace Health Centre
P.O. Box 3070
Halifax, NS
Canada B3J 3G9
Phone: 902-470-8479
Fax: 902-470-8486

Dr. Kevin Farrell
British Columbia Children's Hospital
4480 Oak Street
Room A303, Neurology
Vancouver, BC
Canada V6H 3V4
Phone: 604-875-2121
Fax: 604-875-2285
E-mail: kevin_farrell@telus.net

Dr. Elaine Wirrell
Alberta Children's Hospital
Division of Neurology
1820 Richmond Road SW
Calgary, AB
Canada T2T 5C7
Phone: 403-943-7306
Fax: 403-943-7609
E-mail: elaine.wirrell@calgaryhealthregi
on.ca

Dr. Rosalind Curtis
Hospital For Sick Children
Dept. of Neurology
555 University Avenue
Toronto, ON
Canada M5G 1X8
Phone: 416-753-6057
Fax: 416-753-6046
E-mail: roscurtis@rogers.com

Dr. Jeff Kobayashi
The Bloorview Macillan Children's Centre
25 Buchan Court
Toronto, ON
Canada M2J 4S9
Phone: 416-425-6220 ext. 6276
Fax: 416-753-6046
E-mail: kobayashi@bloorviewmacmillan.
 on.ca

Drs. Daniel Keene & Sharon
Whiting
Children's Hospital of Eastern Ontario
401 Smyth Road
Ottawa, ON
Canada K1H 5L7
Phone: 613-523-5140
Fax: 613-523-2256
E-mail: dkeene@exchange.cheo.on.ca

Dr. Anne Lortie
Hospital Street. Justine
3175 Cote-Ste-Catherine
Montreal, PQ
Canada H3T 1C5
Phone: 514-345-4931
Fax: 514-345-4787
E-mail: lortie.a@sympatico.ca

SOUTH AMERICA

Dr. Luis R. Panico
Mendoza 3373
(3000) Santa Fe
Argentina
Phone/fax:+54-342-4558768
E-mail: dietasur@hotmail.com

Dr. Maria Joaquina Marques-Dias

Professor of Neurology/Child Neurologist

Neurology and Pediatrics Departments

Faculty of Medicine/University of São
 Paulo

Av Dr Eneas C Aguiar 647

05403-900 São Paulo, SP
Brazil
Phone:+11-3069-8673
Fax:+11-3069-8503
E-mail: majomadi@usp.br
Dr. Marcio M Vasconcelos

Av. das Americas, 700 sl 229 bl 6
22640-100 Rio de Janeiro-RJ
Brazil
Phone:+21-2132-8080
E-mail: mmvascon@centroin.com.br

Dr. Andrea Avellanal
Hospital Británico
Benito Nardone 2217
11.300 Montevideo
Uruguay
Phone: 5982-711-91-86
E-mail: cinacina@adinet.com.uy

EUROPE

Dr. Martha Feucht
Universitatsklinik fur Neuropsychiatrie
 des Kindes-und Jugendalters
Wahringer Gurtel 18-20
1090 Wien

Austria
Phone:+43-40400-3012
Fax:+43-40400-2793
E-mail: martha.feucht@univie.ac.at

Dr. Barbara Plecko
University Klinik für Kinder-und
 Jugendheilkunde Graz
Auenbruggerplatz 30
A-8036 Graz
Austria
Phone:+43-316-385-82813
Fax:+43-316-385-2657
E-mail: barbara.plecko@meduni-graz.at

Dr. Lieven Lagae
Kinderneurologie-Epilepsie
Klinische Neurofysiologie
University Hospitals of Gasthuisberg
Herestraat 49
B-3000 Leuven
Belgium
Phone:+32-16-34-38-45
Fax:+32-16-34-38-42
E-mail: Lieven.Lagae@uz.kuleuven.ac.b
 e

Dr. Elina Liukkonen
Helsinki and Vusimaa Hospital

Hospital for Children and Adolescents
P.O. Box 280
Helsinki, Finland
Phone: 011-358-9-4711-4711
Fax: 011-358-9-471-80-413
E-mail: elina.liukkone@hus.fi

Dr. F.A.M. Baumeister
Child Neurology
Kinderklinik und Poliklinik der
Technischen Universität München,
Kinderklinik Schwabing, Kölner Platz 1,
80804 München
Germany
Phone: 089-3068-3352
Fax: 089-3068-3887
E-mail: FAM.Baumeister@lrz.uni-muenc
hen.de

Dr. T. Reckert
Filderklinik-Kinderabteilung
Im Haberschlai 7
D-70794 Filderstadt
Germany
Phone:+49-711-7703-0
Fax:+49-711-7703-1380
E-mail: t.reckert@filderklinik.de
Website: www.filderklinik.de

Dr. Dietz Rating
Dept. Pediatric Neurology
Children's Hospital
University of Heidelberg
Im Neuenheimer Feld 153
69120 Heidelberg
Germany
Phone:+49-6221-56-2334,
ext. 2311
Fax:+49-6221-56-5744
E-mail: Dietz.Rating@med.uni-heidelber
g.de

Dr. Birgit Walther
Teaching Hospital of the Charite
Humboldt University
Herzbergstrasse 79
D-10362 Berlin
Germany
Phone:+49-030-54723539
Fax:+49-0-30-54723502
E-mail: b.walther@keh-berlin.de

Dr. Joerg Klepper
Dept. of Pediatric Neurology
University of Essen
Hufelandstr. 55
D-45122 Essen
Germany

Phone:+49-201-723-2356 or
2333
Fax:+49-201-723-2333
E-mail: joerg.klepper@uni-essen.de

Dr. Viktor Farkas
University Children's Hospital
Semmelweis Medical School,
Budapest
Bókay 53
H-1083 Budapest
Hungary
E-mail: klissz@yahoo.de

Drs. Bryan Lynch and Aisling
Myers
The Children's University
Hospital
Temple Street
Dublin 1
Ireland
Phone: 00-353-86-8197831
E-mail: aislingmyers@hotmail.com

Prof. Pierangelo Veggiotti

Dipartimento di Clinica Neurologica e
 Psichiatrica dell'Età Evolutiva

Laboratorio EEG dell'età evolutiva

Fondazione "Istituto Neurologico
 Casimiro Mondino"

Via Ferrata 6
27100 Pavia
Italy
Phone:+39-0382-380-344
Fax:+39-0382-380-286

Dr. Giangennaro Coppola
Clinic of Child Neuropsychiatry
Second University of Naples
Italy
Phone:+39-81-5666695
Fax:+39-81-5666694
E-mail: giangennaro.coppola@unina2.itb
 r

Dr. Paul Augustijn
Observatie Kliniek voor Kinderen
"Primula"
S.E.I.N.
Postbus 540
2130 AM Heemstede
The Netherlands
Phone:+31-0-23-558800
Fax:+31-0-23-558229

E-mail: paugustijn@sein.nl

Dr. Elles van der Louw
Erasmus MC-Sophia
UMC Utrecht Wilhelmina's
Childrenshospital
P.O. Box 2060
Room SP2434
3000 CB Rotterdam
The Netherlands
Phone: 3110-4636290
E-mail: e.vanderlouw@erasmusmc.nl

Dr. Maria Zubiel
Dept. of Child Neurology
Institute of Polish Mother
Memory Hospital
93-338 Lodz, Rzgowska 281/289
Poland
Phone: 004842-2712080
Fax: 004842-2711412
E-mail: mzubiel@op.pl

Dr. Lesley Nairn
Consultant Paediatrician
Royal Alexandra Hospital
Paisley, Scotland
Phone: 0141-580-4460
E-mail: Lesley.Nairn@rah.scot.nhs.uk

Dr. J.Campistol
Cap Servei de Neurologia
Hospital Sant Joan de Déu
Passeig Sant Joan de Déu, 2
08950 Esplugues (Barcelona)
Spain
Phone:+93-253-2153
Fax:+93-203-3959
E-mail: campistol@hsjdbcn.org

Dr. J. Campistol
Cap Servei de Neurologia
Hospital Sant Joan de Déu
Passeig Sant Joan de Déu, 2
08950 Esplugues (Barcelona)
Spain
Phone:+93-253-2153
Fax:+93-203-3959
E-mail: campistol@hsjdbcn.org

Dr. Antonio Gil-Nagel
Servicio de Neurología
Programa de Epilepsia
Hospital Ruber Internacional
La Masó 38, Mirasierra
28034 Madrid
Spain
Phone:+34-913875250
Fax:+34-913875333

E-mail: agnagel@ya.com

Dr. Oswald Hasselmann
Neuropediatrics
Ostschweizer Kinderspital
Claudiusstrasse 6
CH-9006 St. Gallen
Switzerland
Phone:+41-0-71-243-7-363,
bzw.-111
E-mail: oswald.hasselmann@gd-kispi.sg
.ch

Dr. Meral Topcu
Prof. of Pediatrics and Pediatric
Neurologist
Hacettepe Children's Hospital
Dept. of Child Neurology
06100 Ankara
Turkey
Phone:+90-312-3051165
Fax:+90-312-4266764
E-mail: mtopcu@hacettepe.edu.tr

Dr. Vladimir Komarek
Charles University Prague
2nd Medical School
Vuvalu 84, 150 06
Praha 5

Czech Republic
Phone:+420-2-2443-3302
Fax:+420-2-2443-3322
E-mail: Vladimir.komarek@lfmotol.cuni.
 cz

Dr. Laurence Lion Francois
Centre Hospitalier Lyon Sud
Département de Neurologie
Pédiatrique
165 Chemin du Grand Revoyet
69 495 Pierre Bénite Cédex
France
Phone:+04-78-86-14-95
Fax:+04-78-86-57-16
E-mail: laurence.lion@chu-lyon.fr

Dr. Olivier Dulac
Hopital Saint Vincent de Paul
149 Rue di Sevres
75743 Paris
France
Phone:+33-140-488111
E-mail: o.dulac@nck.ap-hop-paris.fr

Dr. Anne de Saint-Martin
Neuropédiatre
Service de Pédiatrie 1
CHU de Hautepierre

67098 Strasbourg Cedex
France
Phone:+33-0-388127734
Fax:+33-0-388128156
E-mail: anne.desaintmartin@chru-strasb
 ourg.fr

Dr. A. Covanis
Neurology Department
The Childrens Hospital "Agia
Sophia"
Thivon and Levadis
11527 Athens
Greece
Phone:+30-2107751637
E-mail: graaepil@otenet.gr

Dr. A. Evangeliou
University Hospital
Department of Pediatrics
Heraklion, Crete
Greece
Phone: 2810-392329
E-mail: evangeli@med.uoc.gr

Dr. Yr Sigurdardottir
Icelandic Diagnostic Center
Digranesvegi 5
200 Kopavogur

Iceland
Phone: 354-510-8400
Fax: 354-510-8401
E-mail: yr@greining.is

Dr. Björn Bjurulf
Spesialsykehuset for epilepsi
Postboks 53
1306 Bærum Postterminal
Sandvika
Norway
Phone: 47-6755-4000
Fax: 47-6754-5321
E-mail: bjorn.bjurulf@epilepsy.no

Dr. Sergiusz Jozwiak
Professor and Head, Pediatric
Neurology
The Children's Memorial Health
Institute
Al.DZieci Polskich 20,
04-736 Warszawa
Poland
Fax:+48-22-8157402
E-mail:jozwiak@czd.waw.pl

Dr. Nebojsa J. Jovic
Clinic of Neurology and Psychiatry
for Children and Youth

Dr Subotica 6a Street
11 000 Belgrade
Serbia and Montenegro
Phone:+381-11-2658-355
Fax:+381-11-64-50-64
E-mail: njjovic@eunet.yu

Dr. Per Amark
Astrid Lindgren's Children's
Hospital
Karolinska Hospital
S-171 76 Stockholm
Sweden
Phone:+46-8-5177-7026
Fax:+46-8-5177-7608
E-mail: per.amark@ks.se

Dr. Gabriela Wohlrab
University Children's Hospital,
Neurophysiological Department,
Steinwiesstrasse 24
CH-8032 Zürich
Switzerland
Phone:+41-1-266-77-01
E-mail: Gabriele.Wohlrab@kispi.unizh

Dr. Helen Cross
Reader and Honorary Consultant
in Paediatric Neurology

Institute of Child Health and
Great Ormond Street, Hospital
for Children NHS Trust
The Wolfson Centre,
Mecklenburgh Square
London WC1N 2AP
United Kingdom
Phone:+44-207-813-8488
Fax:+44-207-829-8627
E-mail: h.cross@ich.ucl.ac.uk

Dr. Jayaprakash A Gosalakkal
Consultant Paediatric
Neurologist
University Hospitals of Leicester
CDC/Windsor LRI
Leicester LE1 5WW
United Kingdom
Phone:+441-162585564
Fax:+442587637
E-mail: Jay2world@aol.com

Dr. Timothy Martland
Royal Manchester Children's
Hospital
Hospital Road, Pendlebury,
Swinton
Manchester
United Kingdom

E-mail: Timothy.Martland@CMMC.nhs.uk

Dr. Neil H. Thomas
Consultant Paediatric Neurologist
Southampton University
Hospitals NHS Trust
Southampton General Hospital
Mailpoint 021
Tremona Road
Southampton SO16 6YD
United Kingdom
Phone:+44-23-8079-4457
Fax:+44-23-8079-4962
E-mail: neil.thomas@suht.swest.nhs.uk

Dr. Sunny George Philip
Consultant Paediatric Neurologist
Birmingham Children's Hospital
Birmingham B4 6NH
United Kingdom
Phone:+44-121-3338149
Fax:+44-121-3338151
E-mail: SUNNY.PHILIP@bch.nhs.uk

Dr. Ruby Schwartz
Central Middlesex Hospital
Acton Lane
London NW10 7NS
United Kingdom

Phone:+44-020-8453-2121
Fax:+44-020-8453-2096
E-mail: Ruby.Schwartz@nwlh.nhs.uk

Dr. Colin Ferrie
Department of Paediatric
Neurology
Clarendon Wing
Leeds General Infirmary
Leeds LS2 9NS
United Kingdom
Phone:+44-0113-392-2188
Fax:+44-0113-392-5731
E-mail: Collin.Ferrie@leedsth.nhs.uk

Dr. Frances Gibbon
Department of Child Health
University Hospital of Wales
Cardiff
United Kingdom
Phone:+44-29-2074-3542
E-mail: Frances.Gibbon@cardiffandvale.
 wales.nhs.uk

MIDDLE EAST

Dr. Mohammad Ghofrani
Professor of Paediatric Neurology

Shaheed Beheshti University of Medical
 Sciences and Health Services:
Mofid Hospital
Shariati Street
Tehran
Iran
Phone:+98-21-22200041

Dr. Tally Lerman-Sagie
Director of Pediatric Neurology Unit
Wolfson Medical Center
Holon
Israel
Phone:+972-35028458
Fax:+972-35028141
E-mail: asagie@post.tau.ac.il

Dr. Bruria Ben'Zeev
Safra Children's Hospital
Sheba Medical Center
Ramat Gan
Israel 52621
Phone:+972-35302577
E-mail: benzeev4@netvision.net.il

Dr. Generoso G. Gascon
Dept. of Neuroscience, MBC J-76
King Faisal Specialist Hospital &
 Research Center

P.O. Box 40047 Jeddah 21499 Saudi
 Arabia
Phone:+966-2-667-7777, ext.
5813
Fax:+966-2-667-7777, ext. 5819
E-mail: generoso_gascon@hotmail.com

AFRICA

Dr. Simon Strachan
Bedford Gardens Hospital
Paediatric Centre
Bradford Road
Bedford Gardens
Gauteng, South Africa
Phone: 011-493-2613/011-622-2771
E-mail: sstracha@mweb.co.za
E-mail: megawlk@absamail.co.za

Dr. Jo M Wilmshurst
Head of Paediatric Neurology
5th Floor ICH
Department of Paediatrics
Red Cross Children's Hospital
Rondebosch
Cape Town 7700, South Africa
Fax:+27-21-689-2187
E-mail: wilmshur@ich.uct.ac.za

ASIA

Drs. Ada Yung and Virginia Wong
Department of Paediatrics and
Adolescence Medicine
University of Hong Kong
Queen Mary Hospital
Hong Kong SAR
Phone: 852-2855-4485
Fax: 852-2855-1523
E-mail: vcnwong@hkucc.hku.hk
E-mail: ayung@hkucc.hku.hk

Dr. Yukio Fukuyama
Child Neurology Institute
6-12-17-201 Minami-Shinagawa,
Shinagawa-ku
Tokyo 140-0004
Japan
Phone: 81-3-5781-7680
Fax: 81-3-3740-0874
E-mail: yfukuyam@sc4.so-net.ne.jp

Dr. Hirokazu Oguni
Department of Pediatrics
Tokyo Women's Medical
University
8-1 Kawada-cho, Shinjuku-ku

Tokyo 162-8666
Japan
Phone:+81-3-3353-8111
Fax:+81-3-5269-7338
E-mail: hoguni@ped.twmu.ac.jp

Dr. Benilda Sanchez
Head of the Epilepsy Monitoring
Program of Street. Luke's
Manila
Philippines
Phone: 632-723-0301, ext.5452
Fax: 632-727-5452
E-mail: beni779@hotmail.com

Dr. Yong Seung Hwang
Professor, Pediatrics, Pediatric
Neurology
Seoul National University
Children's Hospital
28 Yon Gun Dong, Jong Ro Gu
Seoul 110-744
South Korea
Phone:+82-2-760-3629
Fax:+82-2-743-3455
E-mail: childnr@plaza.snu.ac.kr

Dr. Huei-Shyong Wang
Division of Pediatric Neurology

Chang Gung Children's Hospital
Chang Gung University
Taiwan
Phone:+886-0-968-110264
Fax:+886-3-3277295
E-mail: wanghs444@cgmh.org.tw

Dr. Pipop Jirapinyo
Professor of Pediatrics, Pediatric
Nutritionist
Nutrition Unit
Department of Pediatrics
Faculty of Medicine Siriraj
Hospital
Mahidol University
2 Prannok Road
Bangkoknoi, Bangkok 10700
Thailand
Phone: 662-411-2535
E-mail: sipjr@mahidol.ac.th

Dr. Pongkiat Kankirawatana
Director, Clinical Neurophysiology
Lab
Pediatric Neurology, CHB-314
The Children's Hospital of
Alabama
1600 7th Avenue S.
Birmingham, AL 35233-1711

(information regarding Thailand experience)
Phone: 205-996-7850
Fax: 205-996-7867
E-mail: PKankirawatana@peds.uab.edu

Dr. Janak Nathan Shushrusha Hospital
Ranade Road, Dadar W
Mumbai 400028
India
Phone: 091-22-24446615
E-mail: jsvpnat@hotmail.com

Dr. Hian-Tat Ong
Consultant, Paediatric Neurology and Developmental Paediatrics
Children's Medical Institute
National University Hospital
Singapore
Phone: 065-67724391
Fax: 065-67797486
E-mail: OngHT@nuh.com.sg

Dr. Heung Dong Kim
Associate Professor
Dept. of Pediatrics, Director in Child Neurology
Yonsei University College of

Medicine, Severance Hospital
134, Shinchondong,
Seodaemun-gu,
Seoul, 120-752
South Korea
Phone:+82-2-361-5511
Fax:+82-2-393-9118
E-mail: hdkimmd@yumc.yonsei.ac.kr

AUSTRALIA AND NEW ZEALAND

Dr. Deepak Gill
Paediatric Neurologist
Children's Hospital at Westmead
Cnr Hawkesbury Road &
Hainsworth Street
Westmead
Sydney NSW 2145
Australia
Phone:+02-9845-2694
Fax:+02-9845-3905
E-mail: DeepakG@chw.edu.au

Dr. Mark T. Mackay
Consultant Neurologist
Department of Neurology
Royal Children's Hospital

Flemington Road, Parkville
Victoria 3052
Australia
Phone:+613-9345-5641
Fax:+613-9345-5977
E-mail: mark.mackay@rch.org.au

Dr. John Lawson
Child Neurologist
Sydney Children's Hospital
Sydney
Australia
Phone:+61-2-93821658
Fax:+61-2-93821580
E-mail: Lawson@SESAHS.NSW.GOV.AU
 Dr.
Thorsten Stanley
Senior Lecturer in Paediatrics
Wellington School of Medicine
and Health Sciences
University of Otago
P.O. Box 7343 Wellington South
Wellington
New Zealand
Phone:+64-4-3855-999
Fax:+64-4-3855-898
E-mail: paedtvs@wnmeds.ac.nz

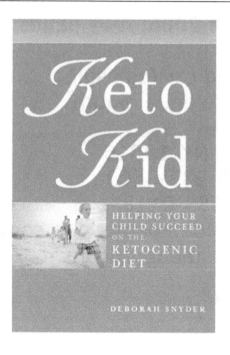

In *Keto Kid: Helping Your Child Succeed on the Ketogenic Diet,* Deborah Snyder, a family physician and mother of a four-year-old "keto kid," provides compassionate advice for parents helping children transition to a ketogenic lifestyle.

Including recipes, time-saving tips, and strategies on dealing with holidays and parties, *Keto Kid* is a practical guide that will enable families to successfully master the ketogenic diet, while making the experience as pleasant as possible for both child and parent.

October 2006, 144 pages, softcover, $16.95

Demos Medical Publishing
386 Park Avenue South
Suite 301
New York, NY 10016
Tel: 1-800-532-8663
Fax: 212-683-0118
orderdept@demosmedpub.com
www.demosmedpub.com

Back Cover Material

One in five children with epilepsy has seizures that are resistant to medication. Even when seizures are under control, drugs may affect children's alertness and mental clarity, impairing their ability to learn and reach their full potential. Many parents are looking beyond currently available medications for a satisfying solution to seizure treatment.

The ketogenic diet is such an answer. This mathematically calculated, doctor-supervised diet is high in fat and low in carbohydrates and proteins, and strictly limits both calories and liquid intake. It helps to control seizures and allows many children to become both seizure-free and drug-free.

This extensively updated edition covers the many advances that have been made in understanding how the diet works, how it should be used, and its future role as a treatment for children with epilepsy. Included is a new section on how the Atkins diet and a modified ketogenic diet can be used as alternative nutritional therapies. This new edition also has an expanded section with recipes and sample meals developed by professional chefs.

The Ketogenic Diet: A Treatment for Children and Others with Epilepsy has been featured on Dateline NBC and in The Boston Globe and various prestigious medical publications. Johns Hopkins referred to Dr. Freeman as "the man world-renowned for perfecting and championing the ketogenic diet" when renaming their epilepsy center The John M. Freeman Center for Pediatric Epilepsy.

Demos Medical Publishing
386 Park Avenue South, Suite 301
New York, NY 10016
www.demosmedpub.com

G

See cream,
Wilder, *50*
Williams story, *183*

X
xylitol, *346*

Z
Zonegran, *21, 64*

CPSIA information can be obtained
at www.ICGtesting.com
Printed in the USA
LVHW021040020322
712307LV00006B/160